CARBS from HEAVEN CARBS from HELL

Discover the Carbs That Tack On Pounds & Those That Don't

DR. JAMES D. KRYSTOSIK

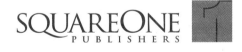

SQUAREONE
PUBLISHERS

The information and advice contained in this book are based upon the research and the personal and professional experiences of the author. They are not intended as a substitute for consulting with a health care professional. The publisher and author are not responsible for any adverse effects or consequences resulting from the use of any of the suggestions, preparations, or procedures discussed in this book. All matters pertaining to your physical health should be supervised by a health care professional. It is a sign of wisdom, not cowardice, to seek a second or third opinion.

Trademarked names are used throughout this book. Instead of using the trademark symbol after each name, the names have been printed with initial caps. This editorial fashion gives credit to the trademark owner, without intention of trademark infringement.

Cover Designer: Phaedra Mastrocola
Cover Photo: Getty Images, Inc.
In-House Editor: Marie Caratozzolo
Typesetter: Terry Wiscovitch

Square One Publishers
115 Herricks Road
Garden City Park, NY 11040
(516) 535-2010 • (877) 900-BOOK
www.squareonepublishers.com

Library of Congress Cataloging-in-Publication Data

Krystosik, James D.
    Carbs from heaven, carbs from hell : discover the carbs that tack on pounds & those that don't / James D. Krystosik.
      p. cm.
    Includes index.
    ISBN 0-7570-0177-7 (pbk.)
1. Reducing diets. 2. Carbohydrates in human nutrition. I. Title.
RM222.2.K795 2004
613.2'83—dc22

2004012778

Printed in the United States of America

10   9   8   7   6   5   4   3   2   1

Contents

Introduction, 1

Part 1

WHAT YOUR DOCTOR WON'T TELL YOU

1. Trust Me, I'm a Doctor, 9

2. A History of Deception, 15

Part 2

THE FACTS

3. The Rise and Fall of Carbohydrates, 37

4. Anatomy and Nutritional Value of Carbs, 45

5. Carbs and Biochemical Imbalances, 61

6. "Battle of the Bulge," 77

7. Fighting Heart Disease and Cancer, 109

8. Diets of the World, 123

Part 3

LIVING WELL

9. Prescription for Wellness, 155

10. Eating Well, 163

11. Beyond Food, 185

12. The 7-Step Knockout Weight-Loss Plan, 191

Part 4

THE AMERICAN-MEDITERRASIAN DIET

13. Prescription for a Healthy Lifestyle, 211

14. Recipes for Good Health, 225

Conclusion, 265

Useful Forms, 267

References, 271

Index, 279

I would like to dedicate this book to my Grandmother Trawinski.
She gave me a wonderful mother: a friend who has always
been eager to encourage me in pursuing my dreams.
My grandmother was not educated, however, she was a wise woman.
One of the things she taught me about health, I'll never forget.
She said, "You can always skimp on the house you live in,
the car you drive, and even the clothes you wear,
but never skimp on the foods you put inside your body."

Acknowledgements

There are several people I would like to thank for making this book a reality. My family deserves many thanks for its support and understanding during the time it took to research and write this book. I want to thank my wife and best friend, Mary Ann, who patiently supported me in pursuing this project. She sacrificed a great deal to allow me to finish this book. Besides her many responsibilities with our six children, she spent long hours proofreading and editing the book. A big thanks to my son Ed, who is not only a great son but a dear friend. His patience and skills are second to none. Besides creating all the graphics in the book, Ed also helped proofread and edit. He is an amazing, multi-talented young man and I could not have completed this book without him. To my other children—Clare, Amy, Jeremy, Andrea, and Bobby—who rarely complained that I spent countless hours on the computer: I love them all dearly and am so grateful for their positive support. To my sister Arlene, my efficient office manager and friend, who freed many hours of time for me to write.

I would like to thank my editors, Mary Ann Krystosik, Yolanda Houdak, Jill Gent, Arlene Rau, and especially Linda Cernjul, for their skills and support in completing this book.

Finally, I would like to thank my patients for teaching me how to appreciate the diversity and sanctity of life.

Introduction

Do Carbohydrates Make You Fat?

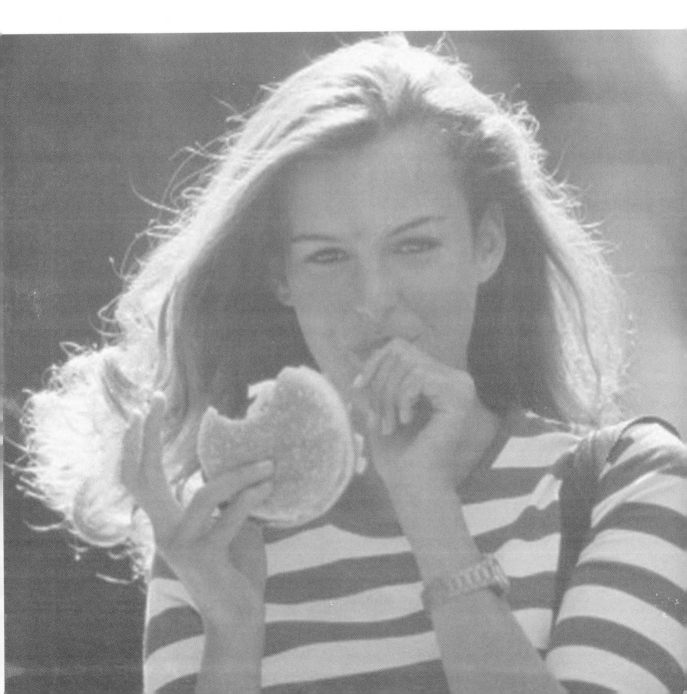

Introduction

Three out of four Americans say there is too much conflicting information about diet. How are Americans making food choices?

—American Dietetic Association

- *What is a carbohydrate?*

- *Do carbohydrates make you fat?*

- *Are low-carbohydrate diets safe?*

- *Do you need carbohydrates?*

- *Do the world's healthiest populations eat low-carbohydrate diets?*

- *Should you eat more protein and fat?*

- *Should you eat more carbohydrates and less protein and fat?*

- *Are low-carb diets based on science or theory?*

- *Does the glycemic index give misleading weight-loss advice?*

- *Does following the USDA Food Guide Pyramid make you fat?*

Do you feel like a pickle-in-the-middle, sandwiched within the confusing debate between low-carb, high-protein diets and those that promote high-carbs and low-fat? Don't worry, you're not alone—millions of Americans are in the same predicament. It's a difficult subject to ignore these days. The number-one food debate in the nation is heating up fast. Are carbohydrates the enemy or the hero in America's "battle of the bulge"?

It seems that just about every other day, you can find a new book, magazine, or news release that adds more fuel to the hottest diet debate of the century. Currently, "carbophobia" is sweeping the nation! This carb-bashing, high-protein diet fad has received a great deal of national attention. And it's no surprise that low-carb diet books are flying off bookstore shelves. It's because they are simply telling people what they want to hear—that they can experience rapid weight loss and improved health while eating large quantities of foods that they have always been taught to eat sparingly: beef, pork, lamb, cheese, cream, and even deep-fried fare.

This latest diet frenzy is challenging decades of advice prescribed by mainstream health experts—eat a high-carb, low-fat diet. Staunch low-carb, high-fat supporters have managed to turn thirty years of solid research upside down. Health consumers are baffled by it all. Considering all the mixed messages we are getting on what to eat, is it any wonder that millions of Americans are confused and unsure of which recommendations to follow? Weight-conscious individuals everywhere are eagerly searching for a permanent weight-loss solution. Is locking the carbohydrates in the kitchen cupboard the answer?

Carbs from Heaven, Carbs from Hell examines these issues and provides practical and safe recommendations to help you choose carbohydrates wisely. As you will see, all carbohydrates are *not* created equal. There are good carbs and bad carbs. So get ready to take the hell out of carbs, and put the heaven back in them just for the "health" of it.

Divided into four parts, this book begins with a section called "What Your Doctor Won't Tell You." The goal of this section is to help you realize that passively following your doctor's advice without question and/or without getting a second opinion may be detrimental to your health—it could even be fatal. No matter how compassionate, competent, or well intentioned your doctor may be, if he or she does not have all the facts, your health may be in jeopardy.

Is your doctor properly trained in nutrition? Is he or she qualified to separate the facts from the myths regarding diet trends? Most everyone knows that the foods we eat directly affect our health and well-being. The big question is: Which health expert has the right formula to help us stay fit and trim? The science of nutrition is young and constantly changing. The reality is that your doctor may have very little training in this area. Most doctors have barely enough time to review all of the new information on drugs, let alone the latest research on nutrition. Even when they do receive nutritional information, the facts may have been skewed by the hands of big corporations, which arguably have little or no interest in your health and well-being. The truth is, many doctors may be just as confused as you are regarding what to eat.

Today's health care consumer must be wise and constantly vigilant. Survival in the twenty-first century requires being prepared to encounter giants. Not the type of giants that storybook heroes face, but the corporate giants, which can be more ruthless than the mythological ones. John Knowles, former president of the Rockefeller

Foundation, stated, "The next major advance in the health of the American people will be decided by what the individual is willing to do for himself."

Mr. Knowles' advice—take care of your own health—is actually the take-home message found in Part 1. It explains the importance of participating in your own health care by taking a proactive role with your doctor, and by making informed choices, including the carbohydrates you eat. To help steer you in the right direction, compelling information is presented that will encourage you to think about the choices you make every day.

In Part 2, "The Facts," you will discover straightforward details about the carbs from heaven and those from hell. From the dawn of civilization to the present day, carbohydrates have made a huge impact on the health and well-being of all societies. Nature has provided a storehouse filled with a variety of carbohydrate foods that are rich sources of health-promoting vitamins, minerals, antioxidants, fiber, and phytochemicals. Its bounty of fresh fruits, vegetables, whole grains, beans, and legumes is an uncompromised source of carbohydrates. Knowing which ones to eat, and which ones to avoid can help you feel great and lose weight—safely and permanently.

The advent of agriculture and the cultivation of grains (carbohydrates) was one of the most important accomplishments in human history. However, the same cannot be said for the modern milling and processing of the noble grain. History reveals that from the time of the Roman Empire, only affluent members of all societies were able to obtain refined grains. It wasn't until the Industrial Revolution that refined grains were available to the masses, which, unfortunately, disrupted the course of the health of the human race. Fortunately, a growing awareness of the value of unrefined carbohydrates is gaining momentum. Let us hope that it continues.

Science is just now beginning to unlock the hidden treasure of the nutrients stored in carbohydrates. In Part 2, you will discover how carbohydrates from heaven have the power to protect you from the ravages of aging, and provide you with a lifetime of optimal health. You will also learn why carbohydrates from hell accelerate the aging process and can lead to a life riddled with illness.

This section also provides an explanation of several diets of the world that are currently competing for public attention. Included are the standard American diet, which follows the guidelines of the USDA Food Guide Pyramid; the diets of Latin America, Asia, and the Mediterranean; and the Low-Carb, High-Protein diet, which is based on a number of the more popular diet plans of this type. I call them the "Good, the Bad, and the Ugly." Soon, you'll see which ones are which.

Part 3 offers a prescription for wellness. You don't have to accept a lifetime of illness. Fatigue, headaches, digestive problems, and muscle aches and pains are not a natural part of the aging process. You can experience a lifetime of wellness without these symptoms, but you must first be able to commit to a lifestyle that encourages it. The "7 Steps to Living Well" show just how easy and how much fun it can be to embrace the principles for enjoying a healthy life.

If you have been bouncing in and out of diets over the years, the "7-Step Knockout Weight-Loss Plan," also presented in this section, will help give you the power to lose weight and keep it off—*without dieting.* That's right. The most refreshing part of this program is that you can lose those unwanted pounds without counting calories or fat grams. Even better, it is a time-proven plan that allows you to eat many of the carbohydrates you like, as long as they are carbohydrates from heaven. I have been using this lifestyle plan successfully in my clinic for the past seventeen years. The key to its success is learning how to reach optimal health, rather than temporarily losing weight to fit into smaller clothes. The natural outcome of good health is a fit and trim body. Find out how you can have your cake, and eat it too—while losing weight without even trying.

Part 4 helps get you off to a healthy start. My American-MediterrAsian diet will show you how. Based on the pleasurable culinary traditions of three of the world's healthiest populations—Latin America, the Mediterranean, and Asia (and a touch of California cuisine)—this dietary plan is truly one without boundaries. By following this intercultural eating style, you can end the obsession of counting calories and fat grams, as well as the guilt that tags along with it. You will experience a new relationship with food—one that will help you develop a connection between food, pleasure, and health. Also presented is an extensive collection of delicious easy-to-prepare recipes, as well as a suggested meal plan. Designed to stimulate the pleasure centers of your mind and palate while contributing to your overall health, these gourmet recipes will allow you to discover the aromas, tastes, and elegant fare of the healthiest cultures of the world.

Simply put, *Carbs from Heaven, Carbs from Hell* presents the truth about carbohydrates—what they are, what they do, and which ones are right for you. Its easy-to-follow, proven strategies will further show you how to lose weight safely and permanently while maintaining good health at the same time.

Part 1

What Your Doctor Won't Tell You

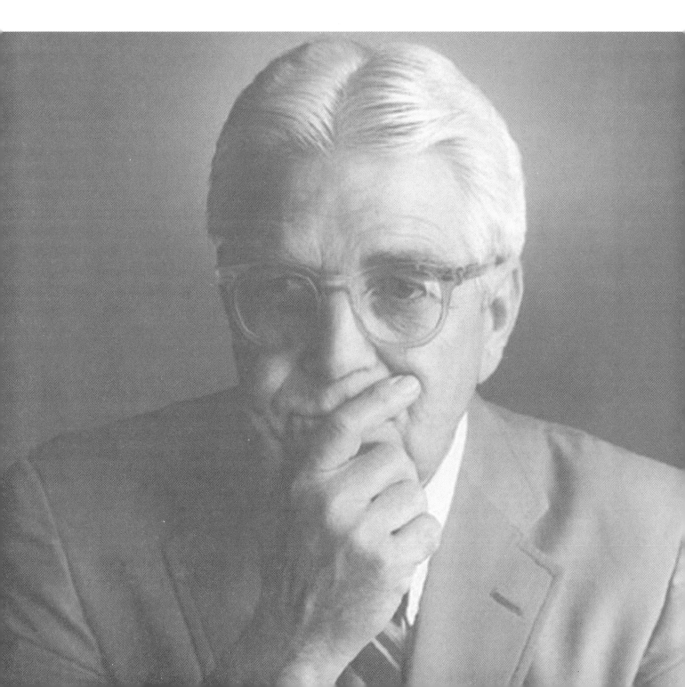

Chapter One

"Trust Me, I'm a Doctor"

Throughout human history, people have placed their trust and lives in the hands of doctors. Although this innocent trust may have been okay in the past, today you had better be more careful. In the twenty-first century, something terrible has eroded the trust we have enlisted to doctors. Corporate giants are now manipulating the guardians of our health for profit. Conflict of interest has penetrated deep inside the medical establishment. When your doctor reads a current medical journal, chances are corporate giants have spun the recommendations for prevention and treatment of disease. According to Meryl Nass, M.D., in an article that appeared in *Health News Analyzer*, "*The Journal of the American Medical Association* reported that a full nine out of ten doctors on committees that develop clinical guidelines had financial ties to the industry whose product they recommend."

Health is one of our most important assets. Consequently, health care choices should be made with careful thought. Wise health care consumers must take charge of their well-being and make informed decisions to protect themselves and their families from health fraud. No one should make a health care decision without first investigating all of the facts and then getting a second opinion. If you don't, you could end up on an operating table under the direction of a surgeon with a hyperactive knife. Or you may end up following the advice of a best-selling weight-loss author that may put your health in jeopardy. Uninformed decisions could have serious consequences.

Who's Afraid of the Big Bad Carbs?

People who are trying to lose weight are one of the most vulnerable targets for health care fraud. Americans are desperate in this battle of the bulge. Consequently, there are many weight-loss gimmicks and diets up for sale. It's hard to believe, but at the present time, there are several diet doctors who applaud the virtues of eating large quantities of artery-clogging saturated-fat foods. Although over thirty years of research has proven that too much saturated fat is harmful to our health, many new diet gurus are still convincing millions of Americans to believe otherwise. These "experts" have capitalized on the insatiable desire of millions of Americans who want to believe that large quantities of meat and other foods that are high in saturated fat and cholesterol are good for them. Many low-carb diet doctors encourage us to fill our plates with bacon, eggs, steak, ham, and whipped cream—without guilt or fear. Is it any wonder that these authors have become so popular and are now America's heroes? Although not all low-carb diets recommend such outrageous amounts of saturated fat, they still insist on turning down the carrots, potatoes, rice, whole wheat bread, and other innocent carbs. Why? Because they claim carbs are to blame for the extra weight Americans are carrying around their waistlines. This new breed of diet doctors has managed to convince millions of Americans to put carbs in the doghouse.

The truth is, you will lose weight on a low-carb diet—temporarily. But not because of some magic weight-loss formula that stems from the various types of low-carb diets. I guarantee you will be surprised when you discover why the weight comes off. You'll also discover that you can lose more than just weight on this type of diet.

Low-carb diets are not as good as they sound. They come with several short-term side effects, and there are no long-term studies to prove they are safe. I'm afraid that this type of diet is not just another craze. This one is a big problem with some serious long-term health risks. A weight-loss plan that claims you can eat as much high saturated-fat food as you want, ought to at least make you wonder if it might be harmful. A diet that restricts the intake of carbs, a food group that humans have thrived on for over 10,000 years, should at least send up a small red flag. Think about the following:

❏ **Low-carb diets are based on unproven theories.**
Proponents of low-carb diets claim that because carbohydrates raise blood sugar levels, they automatically raise insulin levels to the same degree. They claim elevated insulin levels trigger the storage of fat—therefore carbohydrates make you fat. As you will soon see, although there is a grain of truth to this theory, it is only a half-truth that misleads eager individuals into a false sense of why this diet causes weight loss.

❏ **Low-carb diets contradict science.**
Low-carb diets fly in the face of well-researched evidence. There are no long-term studies to prove low-carb diets are safe, but there is substantial data showing that they can be harmful. Research provided by the World Health Organization, the

American Heart Association, the American Cancer Society, and the American Dietetic Association warns of the potential long-term risks of a low-carb and/or high-protein diet.

❏ **Low-carb diet doctors are confused.**

Fad diet doctors conveniently ignore the fact that many world populations eat a high-carb diet, yet they have a low incidence of obesity and chronic disease. These cultures eat more carbohydrates and less protein than their overweight American counterparts, who are riddled with disease. Thousands of well-documented studies demonstrate the benefits of a plant-based, high-carbohydrate, low saturated-fat diet. In addition, scientists have conducted convincing population studies that demonstrate the time-proven plant-based diets prevent disease and prolong life. Unfortunately, low-carb diet doctors by-pass these studies and push their unproven theories.

Right now, America is engaged in a diet war. A band of revolutionary low-carb diet doctors are battling against the high-carbohydrate, low saturated-fat stance of the established medical community. Interestingly, a large portion of the alternative health care community has joined forces with the orthodox medical community on this particular issue. However, it must be mentioned that the alternative health care camp's version of a high-carbohydrate, low saturated-fat diet is much different from the orthodox medical community's version. Unfortunately, many confused, overweight Americans are trapped in the middle of this battlefield. "Should I eat a low-carb, high-protein diet, or a high-carb, low-protein diet?" Currently, the low-carb camp has gained a lot of momentum. Low-carb diet doctors have convinced millions of desperate and defenseless Americans to join their ranks.

Are carbohydrates bad for you? Do they make you fat? These questions need answers that are based on scientific evidence. My intention is to defend carbs from heaven, and prove to you that the right type of carbohydrates can help you lose weight. I will provide plenty of evidence that proves carbs from hell are the real culprit in the fight against the fattening of America. My clinical experience reveals that you can enjoy carbs from heaven without reservation while maintaining a fit and trim body.

Finally, people need to know that the current low-carb diet craze is not a new phenomenon. It is merely a recycling of the discredited and dangerous high-protein diet mania of the 1970s. One must wonder, if it didn't work back then, why would people fall for it again? History has a way of repeating itself—even with unsuccessful and dangerous diets.

Your Health Under Siege

Before I unveil the identity of the carbs from heaven and the carbs from hell, I think you should understand why your doctor has failed to educate you on this important matter. First of all, doctors don't learn about nutrition in medical school. According to Dr. D. DiAngelis, editor of *The Journal of the American Medical Association,* "Physicians are inadequately trained in nutrition." If your doctor was capable of teaching you about the subject of nutrition, you wouldn't be caught in the middle of a low-carb/high-carb diet debate—confused. If your doctor was taught unbiased science in medical school, you wouldn't have to try and figure out how to be fit and trim on your own. The truth is, your doctor may be as confused on the subject as you are.

Health care in America is at a crossroads. Millions of people are now questioning medical authorities on a variety of issues. The general public has access to more information on health than at any other time in history. Consequently, many people are challenging their doctor's recommendations instead of blindly accepting advice that may lead to a future health problem. Sometimes patients know more about specific health problems than their doctors—especially when it comes to nutrition.

There is a large body of important health information that is hidden on the shelves of medical research centers—placed there by the hands of corporate giants. In the next chapter, I will expose several of these medical cover-ups to help you appreciate the magnitude of the health care deception we are all faced with. The take-home message is this: Your doctor is no longer the independent guardian of your health. He or she has become a part of a corporately managed medical machine.

In the following pages, you will discover "unholy alliances" between corporate giants and university research facilities, as well as misleading information disseminated by self-serving interest groups and "health experts." They have misguided and manipulated you and your doctor to help promote the sale of their goods and services. They have reduced the distribution of knowledge to a service for profit.

Consumer Beware

The climate in health care is changing quickly. Innocence and integrity are being replaced by greed and power. Individuals inside corporations and educational institutions manipulate, delay, suppress, and even withhold vital health information—for profit. For many years, consumer advocate groups, and alternative health care providers have tried to warn the public that our health is being threatened by self-interest groups. Important issues like the dangers of hydrogenated oils and artificial sweeteners, the inflammation associated with heart disease, the benefits of vitamins, and the valuable services rendered by chiropractic health care physicians have all been suppressed. The hands of orthodox doctors were tied. They either ignored these issues or told their patients that there was no scientific evidence to back them up. Things are different now. Conventional medicine has been forced to admit the truth. This information, however, has been hidden from the public for so many years, the average person becomes confused when trying to sort through it all. My goal is to help clear up some of this confusion, so you can make informed health care choices in the future.

Right now, government health agencies, your doctor, the food industry, and best-selling authors are all sending mixed messages on the role of carbs in our diet. Whom should you believe? Can we trust the government? Since "Watergate," public trust in the government has plummeted. Can you trust your doctor? You will soon discover that the nutritional advice of most doctors is not necessarily reliable. Most people can see through the propaganda of the food industry. Distrust and confusion has left the door wide open for fad diet doctors to come in and promote their unproven ideas. They have convinced a growing segment of the American population that carbs are the villain—the cause of expanding waistlines, obesity, heart disease, and even cancer. What these diet doctors fail to acknowledge is the overwhelming evidence pointing to the benefits of carbs from heaven in reversing all of these problems.

It is time for a reality check. In addition to saturated fat, carbs from hell are the biggest threat to your expanding waistline. They tack on extra pounds and, at the same time, depress your immune system, increasing your risk for heart disease, diabetes, and other debilitating diseases. On the other hand, carbs from heaven can help you win the "battle of the bulge," while lowering your risk for a number of diseases.

No one can afford to ignore these issues. The consequences are too costly—your health is at risk. If your doctor has failed to inform you on these matters of health, I suggest that you take immediate action to be more proactive in your health care choices. But please, don't misunderstand me. It is not my intention to degrade the noble profession of medical doctors. These men and women have dedicated their lives to the service of the sick and dying, and should be held in great regard. Unfortunately, most doctors are unaware of the control that industry and commerce has imposed on their profession—including the results of much university-based medical research. My hope is that the information in this book will help inspire many doctors to fight back and let truth win. In the final analysis, the health of the American people are at risk.

The "Misinformation Age"

Marcia Angell, former editor of the prestigious *New England Journal of Medicine*, believes that corporate giants have distorted medical research so much that we are living in the "misinformation age." Similarly, Drummond Rennie, deputy editor of *The Journal of the American Medical Association*, asks the rhetorical question, "Why should we care about corporations trying to manipulate or suppress studies by academic scientists?" He goes on to say, "When I go to my doctor, I'm putting my health and my life in his hands. But how can my doctor know the real facts, the best evidence, when sponsors of research suppress, twist, and spin the evidence? Every time a corporate sponsor messes with the data, the sponsor tricks my doctor. Every time that happens, my treatment and the treatment of everyone else suffers."

I encourage you to re-read the above quote. Question your doctor. Read up on any procedure or medication your doctor recommends. Do some research. Make informed decisions—your life depends on it. My primary objective then, is to alert you and your doctor about this unfortunate health care predicament each one of us faces every day. To ignore these issues would be a grave mistake for those who wish to protect their health, and the health and well-being of their family.

> *"When I go to my doctor, I'm putting my health and my life in his hands. But how can my doctor know the real facts, the best evidence, when sponsors of research suppress, twist, and spin the evidence?"*
>
> **—Drummond Rennie**
> Deputy Editor
> *The Journal of the American Medical Association*

To help you better understand the scope of the fraud that exists in our health care system, consider the following example. One of the most far-reaching health frauds of the last century is the introduction of hydrogenated oils into our food supply. The untold suffering and loss of lives because of this artificial "oiling of America" will never be fully understood. Yet even to this day, people continue to risk their health and well-being by consuming foods that are laced with these "phony fats."

The deception doesn't end here. The following chapter provides an incredible, eye-opening look at even more health shams that have infiltrated our society.

Chapter Two

A History of Deception

In the midst of any war, an army that is unexpectedly attacked by its enemy has been "blind sided." This type of sneak attack leaves the ambushed army defenseless, and results in many casualties. In a similar way, when either you or your doctor are given false or even distorted health care information, you have been "blind sided," and your health has been placed in jeopardy. This chapter presents information on many of the ways the public has been misled.

About Hydrogenated Oil

More than likely, a chronic illness or disease, such as cancer, heart disease, diabetes, arthritis, or multiple sclerosis, has affected you or someone you know. Yet did you know that for many years, it was your doctor's advice that may have triggered some of these health problems?

For at least fifty years, doctors have been advising patients to use margarine or partially hydrogenated corn or soybean oil instead of butter. But has your doctor told you that in a recent study reported in *The New England Journal of Medicine,* researchers at Harvard Medical School who studied 80,000 nurses, found that women who ate just four tablespoons of margarine per day had a 50 percent greater risk of developing heart disease than women who rarely ate margarine? What the report didn't mention is that scientists knew about this health risk in the 1950s.

Back then, research scientists warned the American Heart Association that hydrogenated oils in our food supply were one of the primary causes of the nation's heart disease epidemic. In fact, in 1956, Dr. Ansel Keys, one of the authors of the American Heart Association's first dietary guidelines, warned the scientific community that trans fats were a major cause of heart disease. Dr. Keys' warnings were ignored. Already, the manufacturers of hydrogenated oils had a strong influence on public health policy. By 1978, a mounting body of scientific evidence demonstrated that hydrogenated oils were not only a major cause of heart disease, they contributed to neurological diseases, diabetes, and even cancer. Still, this evidence was quietly withheld from the general public.

Despite this threat to public health, oil cartel lobbying groups were able to create advertising campaigns, as well as institute laws protecting the sales of hydrogenated oils. The stage was set. Without restraint, American consumers were ready to be manipulated by emotional advertising campaigns. From 1956 to the present day, public attention, trust, and spending would be influenced by "slick oil" campaigns. With the endorsement of the American Heart Association and the cooperation of doctors across the United States, corporations encouraged our families to switch from butter to "phony fats" made from corn, canola, and soybean oil. Wesson Oil prompted Americans to spread its refined fat across the country with the slogan, "For Your Heart's Sake." Mazola tooted its big horn by saying, "Science Finds Corn Oil Important to Your Health."

*. . . recently, in a study reported in the **New England Journal of Medicine**, researchers at Harvard Medical School, who studied 80,000 nurses found that women who ate just 4 tablespoons of margarine per day, had a 50 percent greater risk of developing heart disease than women who rarely ate margarine.*

Everyone believed the story, including your doctor. Yet, all along, the truth about the dangers of hydrogenated oils was hidden beneath the billions of dollars that were being made at the cost of our lives. Unfortunately, your doctor was "blind sided" by slippery oil cartels that promoted their cheap, but very profitable food-grade oil. Unknowingly, your doctor was giving you advice that actually promoted heart disease, cancer, and other degenerative diseases.

Every day, more and more chemically engineered foods are lining up on supermarket shelves. Highly processed and often toxic, these foods end up on our kitchen tables. Of course we're led to believe that they are safe. It's true that people can eat these "plastic foods" without any apparent immediate visible harm. But are you sure that the symptoms your doctor is treating you for are not caused by one or more of these chemically engineered foods? Do you know anyone who has had a massive heart attack after eating a baked potato with margarine? Of course not. Yet, scientists know that over time, hydrogenated oils can clog your arteries and cause a subsequent heart attack. But don't worry, I'll show you which oils to avoid and which ones are actually good for you.

Hydrogenated oils are certainly not the only toxic food that has found its way into our food supply. Despite repeated warnings from well-respected researchers and consumer advocate groups, many other toxic substances have been allowed on the supermarket shelves. These artificial ingredients should be labeled as poison, yet their manufacturers have received the seal of approval from government agencies, educational institutions, and your doctor. Your doctor has fallen asleep on the job. Doctors, once the "watchdogs" of our health, are beginning to wake up, only to discover that the "fox is sleeping in the hen house."

Artificial Sweeteners . . . Nothing Sweet About `Em!

Would a mother knowingly give her child a poison beverage or a toxic food? Certainly not. Yet, every day, millions of parents give their children foods and drinks labeled "diet" and "sugar free"—foods that may be hazardous to our most prized possessions. Since artificial sweeteners were first introduced into the marketplace, manufacturers have assured the public that they are not only safe, they are, in fact, better for you than sugar. But are they really? Millions of Americans eat foods and drink beverages made with aspartame (NutraSweet, Equal) every day, although millions of others refuse. The controversy over aspartame has been raging for over thirty years. Let's take a closer look.

Aspartame is found throughout our food supply—in over 5,000 foods and beverages. It is in soft drinks, juices, and other beverages, as well as cookies, cakes, pies, and other pastries. How did this controversial substance creep into our food supply?

Americans have a big sweet tooth and the food-processing giants have known about it for a long time. And even though sales of sugary foods have always been good, for years, many health-conscious Americans have tried to avoid them for fear of getting fat. The average Americans had a scrappy internal "ping pong" game going on inside their minds. "Should I eat this high-calorie, sugar-laced food?" (ping) Or "Should I not eat this high-calorie, sugar-laced food?" (pong) Americans were looking for a sugar substitute.

In 1969, James Slatter, a chemist working for the G.D. Searle pharmaceutical company, sat at his desk while trying to develop a new drug for treating ulcers. When he licked his finger to turn the page of his notebook . . . bingo . . . he discovered that the drug was extraordinarily sweet. Little did he know that he was about to unleash a potentially dangerous sweetener into the food supply. Considering this new sweetener was a conceivable drug, it should have alerted him and food manufacturers of its potential harm. However, greed can blind the corporate mind, and this serendipitous discovery resulted in a multi-billion dollar artificial sweetener. NutraSweet (and later Equal) was born—200 times sweeter than sugar, no calories, no guilt, and just a hidden possibility of danger.

Ever since it was first introduced into the marketplace, the safety of NutraSweet has been at the center of a heated debate. Warnings of its potential harm from reputable scientists and government policy makers have been mostly ignored. Dr. Louis Elsas, director of the division of medical genetics at Emory Medical School, warned that pregnant women and infants should avoid the artificial sweetener because it may cause brain damage to the fetus or the infant. In 1974, the original FDA approval for NutraSweet was withdrawn when studies by Dr. John Olney of Washington University found that aspartame may cause tumors in animals.

Despite concerns of its safety, the food industry knew it had a "guilt free" sweetener that would win the taste buds of many—so it craftily persisted for the approval of NutraSweet for seven long years. Just before NutraSweet received an FDA final stamp of approval in 1981, scientific experiments found that animals fed NutraSweet had a high incidence of brain tumors. Interestingly, the study was actually conducted by G.D. Searle, the manufacturer of NutraSweet. It is the same company that the FDA investigated because of "apparent irregularities in data collection and reporting practices." Why would the FDA accept studies by a company that had questionable research techniques, and obvious financial ties to getting its final approval? What is even more frightening is that the FDA made the final approval for NutraSweet based on studies that it knew were possibly fraudulent. To date, there have been no independent studies to examine these important issues.

Neurosurgeon Dr. R. Blaylock, an associate professor at the Medical University of Mississippi, published author of numerous scientific papers and chapters in medical textbooks, and author of the layperson's *Excitotoxins, the Taste that Kills*, summarizes the concerns many well-respected scientists have voiced about the safety of NutraSweet. "To think that there is even a reasonable doubt that aspartame (NutraSweet), can induce brain tumors in the American population is frightening. And to think that the FDA has lulled them into a false sense of security is a monumental crime."

Since 1978, about 85 percent of the FDA's complaints regarding adverse reactions to food stem from aspartame. There are over ninety different symptoms listed in the February 1994 Department of Health and Human Services Report on NutraSweet. They include headaches, seizures, nausea, numbness, muscle spasms, weight gain, rashes, depression, fatigue, irritability, tachycardia, insomnia, vision problems, hearing loss, heart palpitations, anxiety attacks, tinnitus, vertigo, memory loss, and joint pain. Well-respected scientists and physicians have testified before Congress and FDA boards of inquiry that NutraSweet may have serious health consequences.

Many of the foods that contain NutraSweet are labeled "diet" products. Yet there is no evidence to demonstrate that NutraSweet helps to maintain or reduce weight. There is, however, reliable evidence that suggests NutraSweet is an appetite stimulant. R. Wurtman M.D., head of brain science at Massachusetts Institute of Technology, has demonstrated that high levels of NutraSweet cause cravings for carbohydrates. He discovered that this artificial sweetener depletes a chemical in the brain that signals the body not to overeat carbohydrates. Dieters who eat foods with NutraSweet may actually overeat carbohydrates. Instead of solving their problem, they may be making it worse.

NutraSweet is not an essential food. Do you want to risk possible harm to your health or the health of your children by using this controversial sweetener?

The "Whoops!" Factor

Despite the appalling truth about hydrogenated oils and NutraSweet, you may still have confidence that your doctor is a reliable source of all health care information. But maybe you're also beginning to doubt that your doctor is aware of the finagling that goes on behind closed doors. I'm surprised to see how many people choose to stick their heads in the sand on these critical health care issues. I often hear people say, "If something was good or not good for my health, my doctor would tell me about it."

To these people I simply say, "Remember the 'whoops!' factor." If you're not familiar with it, let me explain. Almost every drug or chemical that has been banned was initially allowed in our midst because it was tested and approved for safety. For example, in the late 1950s, the drug thalidomide was allowed on the market for treating nausea associated with pregnancy. Although it had been tested for safety and then approved, a short time later it was abruptly pulled off pharmacy shelves because it was found to cause horrible birth deformities. "Whoops!" Had your doctor warned you or your family about the dangers of the drug thalidomide?

Perhaps you or your parents remember when physicians back in the 1950s claimed that cigarette smoking was good for you. "Whoops!"

Do you remember when doctors tried to convince us that the pesticide DDT was safe? Do you recall the videos of children being sprayed with DDT on playgrounds? It took years of warning by reputable scientists before DDT was finally banned in the United States because it was proven to be a potent toxic cancer agent. "Whoops!" Did you know that American chemical companies are selling DDT to Third World countries to use in their commercial farming? Did you know that we are getting this same DDT back in our food supply through imported produce?

I hope you don't stick your head in the sand and pretend that there's no need for concern about the safety of artificial sweeteners such as NutraSweet. With a little effort, it can easily be avoided. Remember the "whoops!" factor. Many of the scientists (including some in the FDA), physicians, politicians, and consumer advocates who have investigated the safety of NutraSweet, call this cover-up "sweetgate."

Inflammation: The Real Culprit In Heart Disease

"Our entire understanding of what causes coronary atherosclerosis is changing right before our eyes."

—Dr. Paul Ridker, Harvard Medical School

Most American adults are in a constant struggle to maintain or lower their cholesterol levels. But did you know that even if you manage to lower your level below the magic number of 200, you could still be a walking time bomb—a heart attack waiting to happen? Until recently, doctors couldn't understand why more than 50 percent of people who had heart attacks had normal cholesterol levels. We have all heard of someone who received a clean bill of health from the doctor, only to die the next day from a heart attack. Scientists have recently discovered that these heart attacks are triggered by generalized inflammation, which is associated with a number of causes, including infections, arthritis, and obesity.

Don't misunderstand. Elevated cholesterol is still one of the risk factors that contributes to heart attacks and strokes. But researchers now believe that inflammation plays more of a role in the incidence of heart disease than any other risk factor, including high cholesterol levels. Some scientists have known about this problem since the late 1970s, yet until just recently, most conventional doctors knew little or nothing about it. Alternative health care doctors have been warning their patients about this risk factor for many years—twenty years before the average person heard anything about it from the family doctor. Did your doctor tell you about it back then? Or even now?

Fifty percent of heart attacks are caused by the major blockage of a blood vessel to the heart. Once cholesterol and other biological debris accumulate in an artery, causing, let's say, an 80-percent blockage, a small piece of plaque may break off, causing a heart attack or stroke. In the past, this was the prevailing model of the cause of heart attacks. Not anymore.

Recently, scientists have discovered that the remaining 50 percent of heart attacks are triggered by inflammation in the presence of a much smaller artery blockage, let's say about 30 percent. Such a small obstruction cannot be detected by an angiogram and won't cause any symptoms, and yet it may lead to a heart attack. An artery with a small obstruction is not a problem until inflammation enters the picture and triggers a severe or even fatal heart attack. Dr. Paul Ridker, associate professor at Harvard Medical School and one of the world's leading experts on the association between inflammation and heart attacks explains, "It's possible that arteriosclerosis (plaque in arteries), is nothing more than an inflammatory disease, just like arthritis."

It took many years and a major research study to open the eyes of orthodox doctors to the connection between inflammation and heart disease. Dr. Ridker and his associates at Boston's Brigham and Women's Hospital studied the connection between inflammation and heart disease on nearly 30,000 women over an eight-year period. They demonstrated that women with high levels of C-Reactive protein (a marker for inflammation in the blood), had four times as many heart attacks as those women who had a normal level of C-Reactive protein. Through the results of this research, family doctors have finally learned of the association between inflammation and heart attacks. Dr. Eric Topol, the chief cardiologist at the prestigious Cleveland Clinic explains, "I don't think it's a hypothesis anymore. It's proven."

It's hard to believe, but even with all of the evidence, there are still doctors who are hesitant to order this inexpensive blood test because they refuse to recognize inflammation as a primary risk factor for heart disease. Wouldn't it make good sense to have this test done to help avoid a heart attack? Dr. Ridker says, "C-Reactive protein can predict the risk for heart disease fifteen to twenty-five years in the future." Many researchers and doctors believe it is foolish not to include this important test in a routine physical exam. Be sure to ask your doctor about it during your next check up.

Carbohydrates Offer Protection Against Inflammation

Even though scientists have known about the connection between inflammation, nutrition, and heart disease for quite some time, it took more than twenty years for mainstream medicine to even poke a stick at the problem. Yet, back in 1977, Dr. Richard Passwater, a biochemist, researcher, and author on the relationship between nutrition and chronic disease, uncovered the connection between free radicals, inflammation, and heart disease. Free radicals are unstable molecules that are formed as waste products inside the body during normal metabolism. Many more free radicals are created when stress is placed on the body—including stress from infection and inflammation. Dr. Passwater and other scientists discovered that antioxidant nutrients found in fruits, vegetables, whole grains, beans, and legumes are essential for fighting inflammation and heart disease.

Antioxidants mop up free radicals before they damage cells and trigger inflammation of tissues like the blood vessels in the heart. Antioxidants prevent cholesterol from forming harmful plaque—which leads to atherosclerosis and heart disease. They also lower bad cholesterol and raise good cholesterol to further protect the heart. Doctors of alternative medicine have been prescribing antioxidants to their patients for decades. On the other hand, most orthodox doctors knew little or nothing about the ability of antioxidants to squelch inflammation.

What Causes Inflammation?

Let's take a look at how inflammation—a good thing when it helps to fight infections or repair a muscle injury—becomes a bad thing. It can turn the body's defense system upside down, resulting in possible conditions like rheumatoid arthritis or even a heart attack. Our bodies are routinely irritated or injured by infections, traumas, and toxins. When injury occurs, the body is programmed for self-repair through an orderly series of events. For minor injuries, the body quickly removes the damaged cells and restores normal function. However, if the damage is severe, the body will digest the damaged cells, and then initiate the regeneration of new ones. If too many cells and tissues are damaged, a more complicated sequence of events will occur, setting off an inflammatory process.

Inflammation is a normal and essential body process. With the aid of inflammation, the body is capable of fighting infection, eliminating toxins, removing damaged cells, and initiating the repair and regeneration of cells and tissues. Our diet and lifestyle have a huge impact on the outcome of inflammation. For example, eating too much of the wrong foods can stimulate inflammation, which can lead to chronic swelling and pain. Not eliminating or reducing the intake of these foods can lead to the damage of normal cells, tissues, and organs.

During the inflammatory process, the body releases various chemical agents to

Inflammation, Dr. Atkins, and High-Fat, Low-Carb Diets

When Dr. Robert Atkins, creator of the famous high-protein, low-carb "Atkins' Diet," went into cardiac arrest (his heart stopped) on a spring morning in 2002, he was revived and taken to the hospital. It was learned that the episode was caused by cardiomyopathy, a condition caused by an infection (inflammation) that had spread to his heart muscle. Dr. Atkins had been treated for cardiomyopathy for a few years.

Remember, 50 percent of all heart attacks occur in patients who have normal cholesterol levels and no blockages in the coronary arteries; inflammation is the trigger that initiates the heart attack. Inflammation anywhere in the body can cause a small fragment of plaque to rupture in an artery and cause a heart attack. Dr. Atkins' condition was associated with inflammation around the heart, the worst place it could possibly be. Some of the nation's leading cardiologists, including those from the American Heart Association, warn anyone on the Atkins' diet that they are at high risk for a heart attack. Now that the link between inflammation and heart attacks has gained national attention, you would think anyone considering a low-carb, high-protein diet would be scared half out of their boots to even try it—knowing of Dr. Atkins' health history.

Several common factors can trigger inflammation, such as smoking, food additives and dyes, pesticides, processed "junk" foods, deficiency of antioxidant nutrients, diets high in animal protein, infections (including prolonged low-level infections), and diseases that end in the suffix "itis," such as arthritis. This brings me to my next point. Any weight-loss program that does not improve overall health should be suspect of serious fault. In my opinion, this appeared to be the case with Dr. Atkin's health. I believe that his low-carb diet did not provide his immune system with enough fighting power to knock out the infection and subsequent cardiomyopathy.

Considering the link between saturated fat and pro-inflammatory chemicals, perhaps Dr. Atkins would have been wiser if he had switched to a plant-based diet. It might have helped to boost his immune system and reduce his body's inflammatory response.

police the area. Some of these chemicals increase the blood flow to the damaged area, which, in turn, triggers heat, redness, and swelling. Other inflammatory chemicals send out red flags for the immune system to respond to the damaged area. The immune system sends in the clean-up and repair crews to remove any debris and prevent any "little critters" (bacteria, virus) from invading the area. The more serious the injury, the greater the inflammatory response.

The inflammatory process is counterbalanced with the body's own natural anti-inflammatory process. This safety mechanism helps limit the spreading of the inflammation, while protecting normal cells from being injured during the clean-up process. Once inflammation is no longer necessary, the repair-and-regeneration crew moves in to restore cells and tissues.

The normal maintenance of the body requires the constant repair and regeneration of cells and tissues. These processes are synchronized automatically without you ever having to think about them. However, in order for these systems to work efficiently, you do need to cooperate with your body—through diet and lifestyle.

When Inflammation Gets Out of Hand

When everything is running smoothly, the inflammatory system helps maintain order within the body. However, several things can go wrong with this marvelous system. For example, the body can overreact to an injury, causing the inflammation to get out of control. Also, something may activate the inflammatory process unnecessarily.

Remember, when an injury occurs, the body sends inflammatory chemicals into the area to help clean up the debris. It also sends anti-inflammatory chemicals to limit the inflammation and protect normal cells while the clean-up crew is at work in the area. To maintain order, there must be a delicate balance between these chemicals. Diet and lifestyle have a significant impact on this balance. Exercise decreases the inflammatory response. Smoking increases the inflammatory response. The foods we eat can either trigger inflammation or squelch it. The good news is that all of these factors are under your direct control. Each one of us has the power to turn the inflammatory process on or off. The power to squelch inflammation is on your breakfast, lunch, and dinner plates. All you need is an anti-inflammatory diet. That is exactly what I provide for you in Part 4.

Prostaglandins and Inflammation

Prostaglandins (PGs) are local hormones that play a major role in the inflammatory process. The body cannot manufacture PGs. They must be acquired from the foods we eat, just like vitamins and minerals. There are three different families of PGs involved in inflammation: PG2, which promotes inflammation; and PG1 and PG3, which are anti-inflammatories.

Different types of dietary fat are responsible for the production of different types of PGs. For example, a diet high in animal fats (saturated fat), such as beef, pork, lamb, chicken, or turkey, will stimulate the production of the PG2 family of inflammatory chemicals. On the other hand, a diet high in fruits and vegetables, fish, flaxseeds, walnuts and pumpkin seeds (omega-3 fats), will produce the PG3 anti-inflammatory chemicals. Diets that are high in special plants like evening prim-rose, borage, and black currant seed will produce the PG1 family of anti-inflammatory chemicals. These plants can be purchased in supplement form.

Several research studies have found the amount of inflammatory chemicals circulating in the blood is in direct proportion to the amount of beef, lamb, pork, chicken, or turkey in the diet. On the other hand, the amount of anti-inflammatory chemicals in the blood is in direct proportion to the amount of green vegetables, fish, flaxseeds, walnuts, pumpkin seeds, and black currant seeds in the diet.

Inflammatory diseases are common in the United States. Considering Americans eat such large quantities of animal products, and such small quantities of the foods that squelch inflammation, is it any wonder that we suffer with a plethora of health conditions, such as arthritis, inflammatory bowel diseases, allergies, lupus, and multiple sclerosis? With such widespread inflammation, it becomes quite clear why heart attacks are the number-one cause of death in America.

Things That Should Make You Go "Hmm . . ."

For many decades, doctors and their official voice, the American Medical Association (AMA), snickered at anyone who used vitamins. Over the years, countless people had naively asked their doctors, "Should I take vitamins to help prevent disease?" Many of you already know the classic response. The doctors would smirk, roll their eyes, and say something like, "Don't waste your money. All you need to do is eat a balanced diet. Taking vitamins will only create expensive urine."

But on June 19, 2002, doctors had to eat those words when the AMA published a radical report recommending that adult Americans take a good multiple vitamin to stave off disease. Hmm. . . . In the landmark article in *The Journal of the American Medical Association (JAMA)*, Drs. Kathleen Fairfield and Robert Fletcher of Harvard Medical School wrote, "A large portion of the American population fails to get optimal levels of nutrients in the food they eat." This shouldn't come as any surprise since 90 percent of the American population does not even get the minimal recommended five to seven servings of fruits and vegetables a day.

They wrote, "Vitamins also prevent the usual diseases we deal with every day: heart disease, cancer, and birth defects." Hmm. . . . The report also noted an association between vitamin deficiencies, neurological diseases, and osteoporosis (bone loss). Again, Drs. Fairfield and Fletcher wrote, "Insufficient vitamin intake is apparently a cause of chronic disease." Hmm. . . . Although alternative doctors have prescribed multiple vitamins for decades, they have been ridiculed by conventional doctors for prescribing them.

Although the report in *JAMA* is a big victory for American public health, the vitamin wars are not over. There still remains a huge body of scientifically proven benefits of vitamins, herbs, and other natural supplements that is being suppressed by the pharmaceutical industry and other big businesses. Don't forget, the information in the *JAMA* report had been known for decades, yet it was not handed down to the grass-root physicians until recently. You need to ask yourself why your doctor was left in the dark with his hands tied behind his back, unable to pass this vital information to you and your family. More than likely, he or she was passively following the AMA party line, "You can get all the vitamins in the food you eat—vitamins merely create expensive urine." Unfortunately, millions of Americans suffered and died prematurely from heart disease and cancer because most doctors didn't tell their patients that vitamins could possibly help save their lives.

The *JAMA* report discussed the role of B vitamins in reducing toxic levels of *homocysteine*—a major risk for heart disease. This is safe, sound advice, but it came twenty years late. You see, back in the early 1980s, Dr. K. McCully, a physician and research scientist, had already discovered the dangers of homocysteine. He tried to inform the medical community of the ability of B vitamins to mop up this toxin and reduce the risk of heart disease. The medical establishment, however, rejected Dr. McCully's work—in fact, it almost ruined his career because of this pioneering work.

During that time, even though most people were denied access to Dr. McCully's completely safe recommendations, alternative doctors were prescribing daily doses of 400 mcg of folic acid, 20 mg of vitamin B_6, and 200 mcg of vitamin B_{12} to help prevent heart disease. Did one of your family members die of a heart attack during this period? Why didn't your doctor learn about these facts sooner? If you really want to know, just follow the money trail. It will lead you to drug company and food-industry lobbyists, university research departments, and government officials that are all in bed with each other. Figuratively of course.

For over a half a century, alternative doctors have been insisting that vitamins provide good insurance and treatment against heart disease, cancer, and long list of other conditions—including weight problems. Specific vitamins can help stop food cravings, increase metabolism, and help alleviate depression—all of which can lead to overeating and translate into extra fat. What is the primary source of vitamins? Food. Which foods have the most vitamins and minerals? Carbohydrates. But not just any carbohydrates. They must be carbohydrates from heaven. Which is the largest group of physicians who have been recommending patients to eat carbohydrates from heaven, as well as take a multiple-vitamin supplement for the longest period of time? That would be chiropractic physicians—one of the best-kept secrets in medicine.

One of the Best Kept Secrets in Medicine

"The doctor of the future will give no medications, but will interest his patients in nutrition, in care of the human frame and in the cause of disease."

—Thomas Edison

Chiropractors have been educating their patients about the connection between nutrition, weight loss, and disease for over a hundred years. Unlike medical doctors, chiropractic physicians get many hours of training in the field of nutrition during their schooling. Although the chiropractic profession has always led the way to better nutrition, millions of people have been denied access to their services because of the unwarranted exclusion by mainstream medicine. Although most insurance companies now pay for chiropractic services, this wasn't always the case. For many years, chiropractors were dubbed as "quacks" and "unscientific." Sound familiar? Where did this prejudice originate?

On February 7, 1990, Judge Susan Getzendanner, of the United States Court of Appeals, found the American Medical Association guilty of conspiring with other health care organizations for trying to contain and destroy the chiropractic profession. It was a seventeen-year-long legal battle. Wayne Jones, M.D., Director of the Federal Office of Alternative Medicine at the National Institutes of Health from 1995 to1998, summarized the injustice this way, "A federal court found my profession guilty of a prolonged and systematic attempt to completely undermine the profession of chiropractic, often using highly dishonest methods."

The AMA and its co-conspirators used "highly dishonest methods," to destroy a profession that could have helped save the lives of millions of Americans. One of those lives may have been your friend or a family member. The AMA created elaborate plans to destroy the credibility of a health profession that promotes nutrition, spinal manipulation, and other conservative treatment modalities that are in direct competition with drugs and surgery. It created a policy that made it "unethical" for their doctors to associate or even accept referrals from chiropractors. One of their expert witnesses, a physician himself, testified during the trial, that he would prefer to see a patient die before he would be willing to accept a referral from a chiropractor. Hard to believe, but his testimony is part of the court records for all time.

The AMA's Secret Seek-and-Destroy Mission

Part of the AMA's campaign was to destroy the image and credibility of chiropractors in the minds of the American people. Through verbal terrorist tactics, the AMA told its doctors and medical students throughout the country that chiropractors were "killers and rabid dogs," "quacks," and "unscientific cultists." Any M.D. that was not a member of the AMA was threatened with losing hospital privileges if he associated with chiropractors. The following is a summary of the court remarks that clearly demonstrate the far-reaching effects of the AMA's venom.

"Evidence at the trial showed that the defendants (AMA and co-conspirators) took active steps, often covert, to undermine chiropractic educational institutions, conceal evidence of the usefulness of chiropractic care, undercut insurance programs for patients of chiropractors, subvert government inquiries into the efficacy of chiropractic, engage in a massive disinformation campaign to discredit and destabilize the chiropractic profession, and engage in numerous other activities to maintain a medical physician monopoly over health care in this country."

More than likely, this is the first time you've heard these lies and propaganda the AMA spread about the chiropractic profession. Because of its ruthless measures, you have been denied access to one of the best kept secrets in medicine—chiropractic. It's not a secret anymore, if you want to be healthy, team up with a chiropractic physician to be your health coach.

The Art, Science, and Philosophy of Chiropractic

In case you are not acquainted with chiropractic physicians, let me give you the bird's-eye view of this valuable health care profession. Chiropractic is a branch of the healing arts that is based upon the following principle—the health of the spinal column and nervous system are central to our well-being. The science and art of chiropractic is concerned with relationship between the structure and function of the human body, and the restoration and preservation of health.

Chiropractic treatments support the body's inherent capacity to repair itself and maintain health. A doctor of chiropractic is a licensed physician trained in the diagnosis and treatment of disease. Chiropractors are especially trained in physical examination, radiographic interpretation, and orthopedic and neurological testing.

> *"A federal court found my profession guilty of a prolonged and systematic attempt to completely undermine the profession of chiropractic, often using highly dishonest methods."*
>
> **—Wayne Jones, M.D.**
> Director, Federal Office of
> Alternative Medicine
> National Institutes of Health
> (1995–1998)

Chiropractic physicians use the same methods of consultation, physical examination, laboratory analysis, and radiologic examination as any other physician. They provide a careful examination of the structure and function of the musculo-skeletal system, paying particular attention to the spine. If the spine is not functioning properly, chiropractors apply a gentle, controlled impulse to the dysfunctional spinal segment—a chiropractic adjustment. The purpose of the adjustment is to correct minute spinal misalignments, restore motion to the spine, and release nerve encroachment that may be interrupting neurological messages within the body. Once spinal dysfunction is removed, pain is reduced or eliminated, function is restored to the related tissues, and the body is able to orchestrate a normal healing response.

Accidents, sports injuries, stress, and countless other factors can result in small displacements and loss of motion in the spinal column, with resulting nerve root irritation. Chiropractic adjustments restore normal function and mobility to the spine. They reduce or eliminate nerve irritation, inflammation, and pain, and help the body operate more efficiently and more comfortably.

During the time that Dr. Jones was the Director of the Federal Office of Alternative Medicine (OAM), he invited chiropractors to sit on the OAM advisory council. Dr. Jones worked with them to establish a chiropractic research center. He stated, "The sophistication, professionalism, expertise and interest in science I saw (in chiropractors) impressed me." Contrary to the negative propaganda that was disseminated by many doctors and organizations, chiropractic is scientific and should be an integral part of the healing arts.

In addition to receiving many hours of training in nutrition as part of their core curriculum in school, many chiropractors go on to take postgraduate courses of study in the field of nutrition and functional medicine. Functional medicine, which is taught in chiropractic colleges, is the clinical approach I use in my practice. It focuses on proper nutrition and biochemical individuality in the dynamics of health. One of the goals of this science is to improve the function of the patient's organs and systems, rather than merely treat disease (pathology). Improving function allows the body's inherent capacity to heal and repair itself work more efficiently. In other words, improved function provides the body with the healing power it needs. Laboratory diagnostic tests that analyze blood, stool, and other body fluids are used to assess six important areas: digestion, nutrition, detoxification, immunology/allergy, hormone balance, and heart and circulation. The conservative, natural treatments that are rendered result in improved function and the restoration of health without drugs or surgery.

Chiropractic health care is truly a leader in both prevention of disease and the restoration of health. Although prejudices still remain against this branch of health care, which has been scarred and damaged in the past, chiropractors and medical doctors are finally beginning to work together for the best interest of their patients. Many medical doctors and their patients are angry that they were lied to and misled by a greedy and corrupt medical system. Others have started to work with chiropractors in multi-disciplinary health care facilities. Some hospitals are beginning to include chiropractors on their staff.

Times are changing, yet there is still much valuable health information that is being withheld from the American public. I believe the words of one of our visionary presidents, Dwight D. Eisenhower, should always be in the back of our minds, " . . . the right of the individual to elect freely the manner of his care in illness must be preserved." And keep in mind that no one branch of the healing arts has all of the answers. Truth and cooperation are needed now more than ever.

Dr. Jones put it this way, "If you had told me twenty years ago that a time would come when chiropractors and physicians would be working together in common clinics, when they would also collaborate on chiropractic research funded by the federal government, and when chiropractic services would be recommended by medical and national organizations, I would have said you were crazy. Since this is all now happening, it shows how mistaken I, as a physician, would have been." Now that you know the truth about chiropractic health care, I hope you take advantage of one of the best-kept secrets in medicine.

There are good reasons why I have provided several examples of the struggle between the established medical community and the alternative health care community. Many people are changing the way they relate to doctors. Until recently, medical doctors had a lock on all health care information. In the past, even though your joints remained stiff and painful, or you had a chronic skin problem that would never go away, the family doctor was the only person ever considered to diagnose or treat the problem. All that has changed.

We are now living in a super-information age in which everyone is just a few mouse clicks away from a wealth of information on every imaginable kind of health problem. With the advent of the Internet, the divisions between conventional and alternative medicine are quickly vanishing. In a matter of seconds, both sources of health care offer recommendations for treatment on the Internet. Bookstore shelves are filled with best-selling titles that offer both orthodox and alternative medical information, and they're lined up right next to each other!

People no longer view their medical doctors as gods. One study, published in the November 1998 issue of *The Journal of the American Medical Association*, found that 47 percent of Americans have visited an alternative health care practitioner. Follow-up studies demonstrated that a large percentage of these people said they were satisfied with their treatments and would definitely pay another visit to an alternative health care provider in the future. Times are changing, and many people are starting to think "outside the box." People are beginning to seek *all* of the available options before making any health care decisions.

Although a great deal of misinformation can be found in the field of conventional medicine, be aware that it also exists within the alternative field. Alternative medicine has its own share of greedy people, who may care more about their own self interests than the well-being of those who follow their advice. A recommendation coming from someone who practices alternative medicine doesn't automatically make it the gospel truth. My advice? Consumer, beware of false prophets who exist within both schools of medicine.

Beware of "Wolves in Sheep's Clothing"

Be certain that you seek advice from sources that have not crafted lies resembling the truth. Find out if there is controversy surrounding their recommendations. If there is, be sure to carefully study all of the facts before making any final decisions regarding their advice. Remember the "whoops!" factor. Be certain that the sources you rely on base their recommendations on a substantial amount of long-term scientific studies, rather than a few short-term ones that may prove to be inaccurate down the road.

For example, low-carb diet doctors often use anti-establishment language to lure readers into their camp. Many of the people who try low-carb diets have followed standard medical weight-loss recommendations for years, but have failed miserably. It is easy to understand why these people are drawn to the convincing, but misleading arguments made by low-carb diet doctors. Following one of the low-carb diets to win the battle of the bulge, only to discover that several years later you have developed heart disease or cancer as a result, is not logical. Dr. Dean Ornish, an internist and critic of low-carb diets puts it another way, "Lose weight, but mortgage your health."

Good Science Versus Junk Science

Separating fact from myth in low-carb diets is a challenge. The problem is that the average person doesn't have a degree in nutrition and is unable to distinguish good science from junk science. Consequently, many people believe that low-carb diets are based on good science, when, in fact, they are based on half truths that resemble scientific facts. It is absolutely legitimate for the low-carb diet camp to question and challenge the standard medical weight-loss formula. However, if low-carb diets don't agree with established medical science, they should back up their claims with good science. Anyone considering a weight-loss program should not have to abandon science. Science is not owned by conventional medicine. It is a universal tool that must be employed by both conventional and alternative medicine. Good science and junk science can be found in both disciplines. Having said that, I think it is important to recognize that low-carb diet doctors drive home several salient points we should not ignore.

For example, low-carb diet doctors believe refined carbohydrates are one of the primary causes of America's expanding waistline. *Fact.* They feel that Americans are not getting enough fat. *Fact.* The problem begins when they use these valid points, which are backed up with good research, to drive home the other half of their message, which is not based on good science. For example, proponents of low-carb diets claim that all carbohydrates need to be limited because they trigger weight gain. *Myth.* Carbs from hell are the problem. Or they state that you can eat as much saturated fat as you want because it will lower your risk for heart disease. *Myth.* Excess saturated fat is harmful. Monounsaturated and omega-3 oils prevent heart disease. *Fact.* Separating fact from fiction in the low-carb diet is a challenge. You'll find all of the facts clearly presented in Part 2.

Always Question the "Truth"

Through the information provided in Part 1, hopefully, I have challenged you to question old beliefs, and encouraged you to make informed health care decisions. The material that has been provided in this section is significant to the big picture—your total well-being. The primary goal of this book is not just to help you lose weight, but to help you lose weight *without sacrificing your health.* I want you to win the battle of the bulge, while experiencing a lifetime of wellness at the same time.

Part 2

The Facts

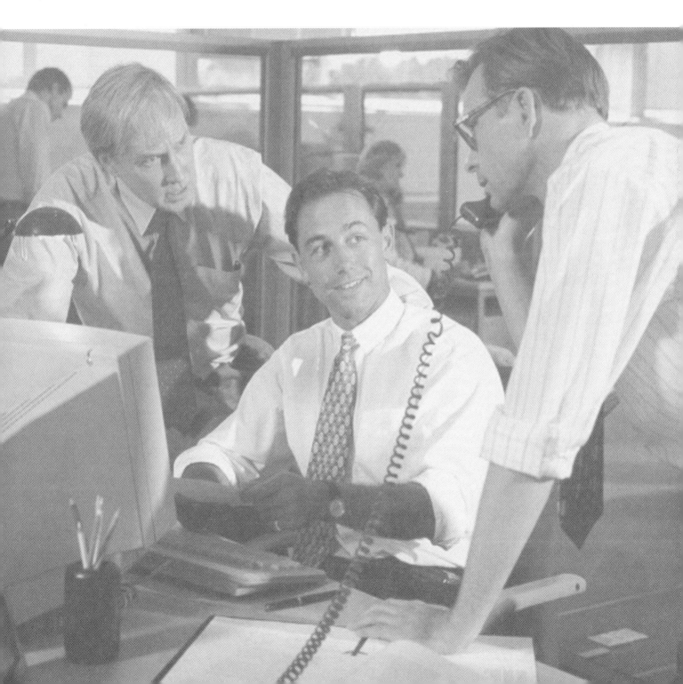

Chapter Three

The Rise and Fall of Carbohydrates

The controversy surrounding carbohydrates is nothing new. Even Adam and Eve labored over their decision of whether or not to eat an apple—a carbohydrate. But the truth is, the apple wasn't the problem—it was the "pair" on the ground! Things haven't changed much. We are still trying to put the blame on carbohydrates, only this time it's not only an apple in question, it is carrots, parsnips, potatoes, and other innocent foods. I don't believe carbohydrates have ever been the problem—the real problem comes from the "nuts" on the ground.

People have an impression that our earliest ancestors were hunter-gatherers. But in reality, early man was more of a gatherer-hunter. Yes, it's true that before the crack of dawn, the brave men of the tribe would grab their clubs and stones while on their way out to hunt for the evening meal. And, of course, the industrious women of the tribe were already busily filling their pouches with berries, nuts, seeds, and root vegetables. At the end of the day, as the men and women sat in their caves eating their collective catch of the day, the women would listen quietly as the men told big fishing and hunting stories from the past. The women would smile, chuckle, and serve a dinner of berries, nuts, seeds, and tubers, along with the "big game" provided by the men: a mole, lizard, or pouch of grasshoppers.

Recent archeological evidence demonstrates that the early human families existed primarily on carbohydrates, probably gathered by the women in a full day's effort. Occasionally, they would feast on some small game provided by a successful hunt. Scientists at the University of Michigan's Human Nutrition Program have been studying the diets of Stone Age people who lived in the Illinois Valley over 5,000 years ago. The examination of their remains demonstrates that these early ancestors ate berries, nuts, seeds, and roots of plants that still grow in the area as weeds. The survival of small nomadic tribes was dependent upon a gatherer-hunter existence—larger populations simply could not thrive on this meager supply of food.

Carbohydrates Spark Civilization

Our ancestors' passage from a nomadic, gatherer-hunter way of life to a settled agricultural-based lifestyle is considered one of the greatest transitions in the development of civilization. This transformation never would have happened had man not developed methods of growing food in an orderly way. Over time, a primitive form of wheat sprouted from the earth in the Fertile Crescent of Mesopotamia. With the help of wind, rain, and the birds of the air, these wild grasses interbred and gradually became a primitive form of wheat called *emmer*. Approximately 10,000 years ago, emmer was harvested, stored, and consumed as a staple in the Mediterranean world. The synergy between man and emmer helped civilization flourish in the Middle East. Agriculture was born, and the cultivation of various crops allowed people to develop large permanent settlements.

As civilizations emerged, every thriving culture cultivated and consumed grains as a staple food. Various grains sprang forth from the earth, adapting to different climates and terrains throughout the world. Wheat and barley flourished in the Middle East. Rice, millet, and some wheat and barley blossomed in China and the Near East. Wheat, rye, and barely grew tall in Europe. Maize (corn), amaranth, and quinoa grew vigorously in North and South America. Barley, sorghum, and millet proliferated in Africa.

Most people in these regions of the world relied on a diet of grains, legumes, fruits, and vegetables, and, to a lesser extent, meat. Those who took exception to this frugal peasant diet were of the smaller wealthy upper class, whose diet often included much more meat. As civilizations continued to flourish, the gatherer-hunters either remained small or vanished.

The cultivation of grain has played an integral part in the cultural history of mankind. In fact, the origin of the word "culture" is derived from the word cultivation. Since the dawn of civilization, cereal grasses, also known as grains, have been the foundation of the human diet. From the dawning of man to the time just before grain was cultivated, it is estimated that the population of the earth was less than 3 million. After the introduction of farming and the cultivation of grains, many thousands of years ago until the time of Christ, the population of the earth rose to about 300 million. Truly, the shift from the nomadic tribes to settled habitation and agriculture marks one of the greatest advancements of human civilization.

Throughout history, grains have played a significant role in the development of civilization. Homer talked about them. The Egyptian pyramid builders survived on them. Jesus fed the multitudes with them. Roman emperors placated the masses with them. Great armies relied upon these carbohydrates for their sustenance. Roman soldiers lived on a diet consisting almost entirely of grains—bread, wheat porridge, beans, cheese, and a little wine to wash it down. Some historians believe the Roman soldier's diet was actually simpler, including only bread and water. Bread was considered the only food "fit for a soldier." It was "hard food for hard men."

Bread, an All-Time Favorite

Porridge—whole or cracked grains mixed with water—and flat cakes were fore-runners of bread. Even in modern times, people continue to eat porridge and various flat breads, which come in the form of pita bread, pancakes, crepes, tortillas, and, of course, pizza.

The first true breads are believed to have originated in the Middle East about 2500 BC. During that time, fermented dough (sourdough) was added to flat cakes to make them rise. At first, dough was baked on hot rocks or griddles, and then it was baked in domed pots made of clay. Eventually, bread molds and ovens were created to improve the rising action of the dough and cook the bread more evenly. The Ancient Egyptians baked their bread in ovens, in which the molds were stacked on top of one another. The Assyrians baked the dough in sealed clay pots that were buried in heated pits in the ground.

Historians credited the ancient Greeks for the development of bread making into an art. By 300 AD, the Greeks had created over seventy varieties of bread. They introduced bread making to Gaul, the area eventually controlled by the Romans. As the Roman Empire expanded, the Greek bread-baking tradition spread throughout Europe. Although porridge and flat breads remained a part of the ancient world, baked breads took a central role in the diet. Every culture has some form of bread—people from every part of the world have been breaking bread with family and friends for thousands of years.

Technology Breaks the "Staff of Life"

Both whole wheat bread (a carb from heaven) and white bread made from refined wheat (a carb from hell) have been enjoyed by civilizations for thousands of years. Wheat was used by ancient Egyptian civilizations to make whole wheat bread. White bread was available during the time of the Roman Empire, but enjoyed only by the wealthy or used during religious celebrations. This changed during the Industrial Revolution.

As wheat became more available, lighter refined breads were associated with the upper class and city dwellers, while dark, coarse breads were connected to the working class and those living in the countryside. During times of famine, disease, and war, milled grains became less available, and even the wealthy were forced to eat the darker, unrefined breads. Psychologically, this may well be why lighter, more refined breads are typically preferred during times of peace and prosperity.

During the Industrial Revolution, the invention of farm machinery dramatically increased grain production, changed the milling process, and caused a rise in the production of refined bread products. For the first time in history, white bread became available to everyone. Soon, whole grain flour was replaced by bleached and enriched flour, which is stripped of most of its fiber, vitamins, minerals, and other natural plant nutrients. Eventually, food processors began adding hydrogenated oils, preservatives, and other chemicals. Today's commercial breads barely resemble the staple food of our ancestors. Technology has broken "the staff of life."

Bread is not the only food that has been losing vitamin power from the farm to the kitchen table. Pasta, cereals, baked goods, and other products made from refined grains have all been stripped of their life-giving elements. They have replaced the whole grain foods that civilizations have relied upon for thousands of years. Manufacturers have managed to mass-produce foods that look and taste good, but are missing one important ingredient—good nutrition.

America has become a nation in which few people go hungry, yet the population is undernourished. The loss of essential nutrients in our diet has caused much unnecessary suffering and an overweight population. It is no wonder that so many people are turning to fad diets that promise miracle cures—promises they cannot keep. These diets are doomed to fail because typically they restrict many important foods that contain essential nutrients, which prevent disease and help maintain a fit and trim body.

Traditional Diets versus "Westernized" Diet

Throughout history, societies have relied on a grain and plant-based diet with small amounts of meat. Carbohydrates like fruits, vegetables, grains, beans, and legumes have formed the traditional dietary foundation of several regions of the world. Since the 1950s, scientists have shown a great deal of interest in the diets of three of these cultures: the Mediterranean, Asia, and Latin America. Based on their research, scientists generally agree that the exceptionally low rate of chronic diseases, coupled with an increased lifespan of the people living in these regions is due to their traditional diets.

Sadly, over the last couple of decades, the rapid economic development of these populations has slowly begun to erode their plant-based way of eating, giving way to a more "Westernized" refined-carbohydrate diet with a dramatic increase in saturated fats. As a consequence, these countries have seen a marked rise in obesity and death rates due to heart disease and cancer. Their scientists have made strong government recommendations to restore the plant-based high-carbohydrate, low-fat diets to help stop the spreading epidemic of obesity and chronic disease. In view of these facts, why would anyone want to risk his or her health by following a low-carb, high-protein diet?

Our bodies need carbohydrates, regardless of what low-carb diet doctors claim! Without carbs, the body will convert protein or fat into glucose—a carbohydrate. And this conversion process is difficult. Besides, most people are big fans of carbohydrates. Who doesn't enjoy the smell and taste of a fresh baked loaf of bread, a piping hot stack of pancakes with maple syrup, or a home-baked apple pie? Restricting carbohydrates is not a normal behavior pattern. I believe restricting or eliminating them from the diet is both physically and emotionally unhealthy.

You don't have to restrict carbohydrates to lose weight and feel great. The eating strategy outlined in this book allows you to eat familiar foods—even most of your favorite carbohydrate foods. But instead of preparing them with refined carbs, I'll teach you how to make them with unrefined ones.

Not All Carbohydrates Are Created Equal

Low-carb diet doctors want you to believe carbs are bad for your health and a threat to your waistline. They claim we need to restrict the amount of carbohydrates we eat in order to tip the scales in favor of weight loss. The truth is, what's most important is the *quality* of the carbohydrates we eat, not the *quantity*. Fruits may be high in sugar, but they certainly should not be lumped together with chocolate candy bars. Fruits are carbohydrates from heaven, chocolate candy bars are carbohydrates from . . . and each will have a different effect inside the body.

Research scientists at Harvard University have discovered that individuals who eat a diet that is high in unrefined carbohydrates significantly decrease their risk for diabetes and heart disease. Those whose diets are high in refined carbohydrates more than double their risk for heart disease. Dr. Gerald Reaven, a research scientist from Stanford University, has studied the link between diabetes and heart disease for some time. He has discovered that refined carbohydrates and saturated fats are linked to a harmful condition he calls *Syndrome X*, which is discussed in detail in Chapter 7.

Despite what low-carb diet doctors would like you to believe, the problem is not the carbohydrates. The real problem is when good carbohydrates turn bad—when a heart-healthy potato is turned into an artery clogging French fry, for example. Throughout history, potatoes have been a staple food in many parts of the world. They actually promote weight loss and good health, as long as you don't fry them, and you eat them in their entirety, skin and all. When the potato skin is tossed out, the fiber and most of the nutrients are lost, and only the fat-promoting starch remains. When left on its own, the starch is absorbed almost as fast as white sugar, and the extra calories turn into fat. A potato without the skin quickly becomes a carbohydrate from hell and an enemy in the battle of the bulge.

My goal is to help you understand the difference between carbs from hell and carbs from heaven. Once you recognize the difference, you will be able to eat most of your favorite carbohydrates. Avoiding carbs from hell will not only help you get rid of food cravings and lose weight, it will also help increase energy and boost your immune system to fight disease. Take advantage of the benefits of carbs from heaven. They will help you keep the weight off, and enable you to enjoy the wonderful tastes and pleasures of all your favorite foods without compromising your health.

Separating the Wheat from the Chaff

Trying to sort out the the good carbs from the bad carbs can be a difficult task—but not as hard as you might think! The "get real" rule is the first thing you should consider when buying carbohydrates. If a food comes packaged by nature, you can be pretty sure that it is safe and good for you. All fruits and vegetables that are still in their natural packaging from the vine or a tree are good for you. But when any of these foods have been processed—cut, peeled, sliced, diced, cooked, fried, dipped in sugar water, or contain preservatives or other artificial ingredients—they may end up causing a lot of trouble. Like some good-looking bad guys, processed foods often present themselves with good-looking exteriors that don't reflect what is inside! The only way to know if the food you are going to eat is good for you is by purchasing it fresh, or by reading ingredient labels

Food manufacturers frequently use deceptive advertising promotions. Bread often comes in attractive packaging that advertises the product inside is made of "whole wheat" or includes "seven grains." Although this may sound pure and wholesome, it could literally mean that the company used as little as 1-percent whole wheat flour, with refined white flour making up the remaining 99 percent. From a legal standpoint, this can be considered whole wheat bread. Crackers often fall into this "shamful" category as well. The outside of the box may advertise "vegetable" crackers or "wheat" crisps, but the vegetables and whole wheat are often the last items on the ingredient list, usually after sugar. And pastas are usually made from refined wheat flours.

Knowing where a food comes from is also important. I don't mean that you should recognize that Hershey's chocolate comes from Hershey, Pennsylvania. I mean that you should know if the food you are about to eat comes from a farm or from a food manufacturer that processes natural foods so much that even rodents eat them as a last resort. Processed foods with long lists of ingredients that you can't even pronounce are a clue to stay away from them. It's likely that the more processed foods you eat, the less fruits and vegetables you'll eat—foods that will help you feel better and lose weight. I'm not telling you to turn away from pasta, crackers, and bread, just make sure their ingredient labels state, "made with 100-percent whole grains."

Chapter Four

Anatomy and Nutritional Value of Carbs

I would like to begin this chapter by reviewing some basic information about carbohydrates—the body's primary source of fuel. Carbohydrates are literally created out of thin air. The building blocks of carbohydrates are carbon dioxide and water, two of the most abundant elements on the earth. When molecules of carbon and water in the air hook up, a carbohydrate is formed. The word *carbohydrate* is derived from this chemical reaction—*carbo* represents carbon, and *hydrate* literally refers to the addition of water.

All of the body's activities from thinking to walking require energy, which comes from the food we eat. Choosing the right type of fuel to run the body is important for maximum performance, and carbohydrates provide a clean source of energy. After the body burns a calorie of carbohydrate, energy is released, leaving the waste products of carbon dioxide and water (the two ingredients that formed the carbohydrate in the first place) behind. This process demonstrates a perfect circle of life, efficient and in harmony with nature's plan.

Our body's energy system is driven by calories. Carbohydrates, protein, and fat are the three primary sources of dietary calories. Both carbs and protein supply the body with four calories per gram. Fat, on the other hand, supplies nine calories per gram. Although protein and fat can be used as fuel to run the body, they are less efficient than carbohydrates, and they leave behind harmful waste products. On the other hand, carbohydrates are a clean and efficient source of fuel, much like propane. Trying to run the body on protein or fat is like burning coal for energy— a less efficient and dirtier source of fuel than gas.

All foods derived from plants contain carbohydrates. Unprocessed fruits, vegetables, grains, beans, legumes, and nuts contain both digestible and indigestible carbs. *Digestible carbs* (starch) can be processed and absorbed by the human digestive system, turned into calories, and used as fuel. *Indigestible carbs* (fiber) cannot be absorbed and do not add any calories to your diet. Friendly bacteria in the gut, however, convert fiber into an important fuel for the intestines.

Zero Calories or Empty Calories?

Since dietary fiber is an indigestible carbohydrate and cannot be absorbed by the human digestive tract, it has zero calories. Fiber can, however, help you lose weight, lower cholesterol and blood pressure, balance sugar levels, and reduce your risk for many diseases, including cancer. With the exception of dairy products, which contain the digestible carbohydrate *lactose,* carbs from heaven are plant-based foods provided by nature. Plant-based carbs are a rich source of vitamins, minerals, amino acids, essential fatty acids, and phytochemicals (chemicals produced by plants that have many health-related benefits). Nature has provided these carbs with more nutrition and fewer calories than any other food, including protein and fat.

Everyone except food manufacturers know that you can't fool Mother Nature. These culprits disregard nature. Most conventionally processed carbohydrates have been altered to the point that they are void of a significant portion of their nutrition. They are also higher in calories, and can cause a myriad of health consequences. In other words, food processors have turned natural health-promoting carbs from heaven into carbs from hell. That's why many nutritionists refer to these processed foods as dead or empty calories. Having an unusually high starch content, these denatured foods have been stripped of their fat-blocking fiber—two big reasons that carbs from hell are a major cause of weight gain. Any nutrients that may remain are insignificant to overall health.

Carbs from hell are all around us. They are in foods like white sugar, white flour, white rice, corn syrup, high-fructose corn sweeteners, and sugar-laden drinks, candy, and snacks. And they are readily available. You can buy them just about anywhere, from supermarkets and shopping malls to school cafeterias and gas stations. Because carbs from hell are so convenient, it's easy for people to eat them.

Carbs from heaven, on the other hand, are harder to find. Although supermarkets may carry some fresh fruits, vegetables, beans, legumes, and a few whole grain breads and cereals, it is the health food stores that carry wider varieties. Their shelves are stocked with carbs from heaven, including organic produce; whole grain breads, baked goods, cereals, and crackers; and prepared meals. Fortunately, as people have become more health-conscious than in the past, several national and regional grocery chains have added health food sections to their stores. Primarily, however, it is health food stores that remain the best places to purchase these foods. The problem is that the average person doesn't go out of his or her way to shop at health food stores.

If you're caught in the junk food spider web, breaking away won't be easy. Liberation from its bondage, however, will empower you with health and a fit and trim body. Knowing the difference between good carbs and bad carbs is one of the first things you'll need to enter the world of good health. The checklists on the following pages provide a listing of both.

Simple or Complex?

All carbohydrates are made from the same three elements—carbon, hydrogen, and oxygen. They are labeled *simple* or *complex,* according to the order in which these three elements are arranged. Simple carbs have a simple arrangement, like a straight line. Complex carbs have a complicated arrangement, like a branch on a tree. The big difference between the two is how they are digested. Simple carbs digest quickly and cause a quick spike in blood sugar levels. Complex carbs digest slowly, and provide a slow, steady release of sugar into the bloodstream.

Carbohydrates can be further classified, depending on whether they are packaged by nature or processed by food manufacturers. Simple carbs are packaged in two ways: *natural, unrefined,* which includes products like honey and pure maple syrup; and *processed, refined,* which includes products like white table sugar and corn syrup. The word "natural" or "unrefined" means the product has been untouched by food manufacturers and contains all of its vitamins, minerals, enzymes, fiber, and other essential nutrients. "Refined" indicates the end product has been tampered with by food processors. The refining process removes most of the essential nutrients, resulting in a denatured food that creates chemical imbalances inside the body. However, it enables these foods to sit on the shelves for longer periods of time without spoilage and/or to serve as cheap ingredients for other prepared foods.

Complex carbohydrates come in the same two varieties as simple carbs. Natural, unrefined varieties include foods like whole wheat, corn, brown rice, and beans. They are the perfect foods for maintaining ideal levels of blood sugar, cholesterol, and body weight because they are rich sources of fiber. This slows down the emptying of carbs from the stomach, while preventing a sudden surge of insulin from the pancreas. In addition, the thick, sludge-like fiber slows the movement of sugar as it makes its way across the intestinal tract and into the bloodstream. The final outcome is a gradual rise in blood sugar. Cholesterol binds to the fiber and is trans-

Carbs from Heaven Checklist

The following foods provide the body with the right type of carbohydrates. For more suggestions and recommended brands, see the Shopping List in Chapter 13.

❑ **Vegetables.** Fresh vegetables are low in calories and high in fiber, vitamins, minerals, antioxidants, and phytochemicals. Includes lots of dark green leafy lettuces, as well as spinach, kale, Swiss chard, mustard greens, broccoli, cauliflower, tomatoes, potatoes, eggplant, bell peppers, corn, peas, green beans, cucumbers, radishes, onions, carrots, beets, and parsnips.

❑ **Fruits.** Fresh fruit provides a sense of fullness and a bounty of flavors. These carbs from heaven are rich in vitamins, antioxidants, minerals, fiber, and phytochemicals. Consider adding them to your breakfast or enjoying them as snacks or dessert. A splash of lemon offers added zing to certain beverages and dishes. Includes all fresh fruits, including berries and melon varieties.

❑ **Beans and Legumes.** These heavenly carbs are rich sources of vitamins, minerals, phytochemicals, and water-soluble fiber, which are needed to maintain normal blood sugar levels, cholesterol levels, and proper weight. And there is a wide variety from which to choose. Includes black beans, black-eyed peas, garbanzo beans, kidney beans, lentils, lima beans, navy and other white beans, pinto beans, split peas, and soybeans.

❑ **Whole Grains.** Whole grains are high in fiber, vitamins, minerals, and phytochemicals. They are filling, low in calories, and satisfy hunger for long periods. The most common grain varieties include oats, corn, brown rice, barley, wheat, and rye; they are available in breakfast cereals, breads, and pasta.

❑ **Milk Products.** All dairy products should be used sparingly. However, when using them, select those made from sheep or goat's milk. These milk varieties are closest in chemical composition to mother's milk. Use cow's milk products cautiously, sparingly. Many people have hidden allergies to cow's milk, which can result in a variety of side effects, including weight gain. Food allergies are triggered by the protein in the offending food. Choose goat and sheep-milk cheeses such as chevre, feta, manchego, kasseri, and Roquefort. Products made from soy milk and rice milk are good substitutes for cow's milk products. However, be certain these cheese substitutes do not contain caesin, a cow's milk protein.

❑ **Convenience Packaged Foods.** Packaged fresh or frozen foods can be heavenly if they are made with 100-percent whole grains, vegetables, and fruits—and contain no refined sugars, sugar substitutes, colors, or additives.

❑ **Sweet Treats and Snack Foods.** As long as they are enjoyed on an occasional basis, certain snacks are delicious healthy foods. Includes cookies, cakes, pies, and other snack foods made with 100-percent whole grain pastry flours, unrefined sugars, real fruit or spreads, and soy or rice milk products.

❑ **Fruit Juices and Beverages.** Since fruit juices are high in natural sugar, drink them sparingly. Includes 100-percent unfiltered fruit juices and fruit-juice sodas with no added sweeteners. Fresh-squeezed juices may be used more liberally.

❑ **Sweet Spreads and Condiments.** Since these products are high in natural sugar, use them sparingly. Includes 100-percent real-fruit spreads and jellies, maple syrup, brown rice syrup, molasses, date sugar, and Succanat sugar, which, unlike their highly refined counterparts, contain vitamins, minerals, and antioxidants.

Carbs from Hell Checklist

The following foods provide the body with the wrong type of carbohydrates. You don't have to give up these foods—simply replace them with wholesome counterparts. See the Healthy Indulgences in Chapter 13 for healthy alternatives.

❐ **Vegetables.** Vegetables from heaven that are fried or overcooked, or that contain refined sugar, artificial sugar substitutes, artificial food coloring, or preservatives, can quickly turn into a carb from hell. (French fries may look like food, but they don't belong in the body.) Fried foods are high in toxins, hydrogenated fat, and calories. Processed vegetables lack vitamins, minerals, and enzymes. Includes vegetables that are fried, overcooked, or canned.

❐ **Fruits.** Any fruit from heaven that is heated to high temperatures and packed in syrup, or contains a sugar substitute, food coloring, or preservatives becomes a carb from hell. Processed fruits have fewer vitamins and minerals than fresh varieties; they also have additional calories due to their refined sugar content. Includes canned fruits, especially those packed in heavy syrup and dietetic varieties, which contain artificial sweeteners.

❐ **Beans and Legumes.** Heavenly beans and legumes that contain hydrogenated oil, salt, refined sugars, food colorings, or preservatives, have been transformed into carbs from hell. They have fewer nutrients and added calories due to their refined sugar content. Includes most canned varieties.

❐ **Grains.** Any processed grain from heaven is a carb from hell. Most packaged products made from refined grains also contain refined sugar, artificial sugar substitutes, hydrogenated oil, food coloring, and/or preservatives. Includes white bread, white rice, white pasta, and most commercial snack foods and breakfast cereals.

❐ **Milk Products.** Dairy products made with refined white sugar, hydrogenated fats, artificial sweeteners, and food colorings may taste devilishly good, but don't be fooled. These carbs are straight from hell. Includes ice cream, whipped cream, dairy powders, yogurt, butter, and cheese. Most harmful are cow's milk products.

❐ **Convenience Packaged Foods.** Prepared dishes that are made with refined white flour, sugar, salt, hydrogenated fats, and artificial ingredients are carbs from hell. They are deficient in fiber, vitamins, minerals, and phytochemicals, and typically offer short-term satisfaction, resulting in hunger rebound. Includes most packaged frozen dinners and entrées.

❐ **Sweet Treats and Snack Foods.** When made with processed flour, sugar, artificial sweeteners, hydrogenated oils, food coloring, and/or preservatives, these foods are carbs from hell. High in nutritionally empty calories, they trigger cravings for more of the same. Includes most commercial baked goods, candies, and sweet packaged snacks.

❐ **Fruit Juices and Beverages.** Many commercial fruit juices and other beverages are highly processed—made from concentrates, man-made chemicals, or both. They contain fructose, corn syrup, or artificial sugar substitutes, as well as preservatives and food colorings. Filled with empty calories, these beverages stimulate hunger. Includes most bottled or canned juices, carbonated soft drinks, and a number of so-called "power" drinks.

❐ **Sweet Spreads and Condiments.** Processed fruits packed in sugar, corn syrup, fructose, or artificial sweeteners, and have added flavorings and artificial coloring are carbs from hell. Unlike natural fruit spreads, these products are higher in calories. Includes commercial jellies, jams, and preserves.

ported out of the body in the stool. Fiber is a drug-free solution for the treatment and prevention of such conditions as heart disease, diabetes, and obesity.

Processed, refined complex carbohydrates include items like white flour, white rice, and noodles. When these refined carbs enter the intestines, trouble begins. Have you ever heard the saying, "The whiter the bread, the sooner you're dead"? The scant amount of fiber in refined carbs enables the sugar to move quickly into the blood (there isn't enough fiber to slow its movement). This results in a sudden surge in blood sugar, which translates into unstable levels. Diabetes, weight gain, and a plethora of health problems can result. Anyone who eats mostly carbs from refined products is asking for trouble. It is important to know if a carb is simple or complex, refined or unrefined—your health depends upon it.

The Anatomy of a Carbohydrate from Heaven

All grains, whether barley, wheat, corn, rice, or other cereal grasses, have the same basic anatomy. They are made up of three parts—the bran, endosperm, and germ. Some grains also have a hull. The physical structure of an unrefined grain of barley is found below.

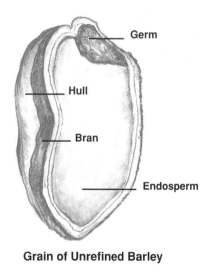

Grain of Unrefined Barley

❒ **Endosperm.** The starchy portion of the grain that provides energy and a small amount of protein and fiber.

❒ **Germ.** The embryo of the plant. It is very rich in vitamins, minerals, and other nutrients to aid the seed while it grows and develops.

❒ **Bran.** The outer indigestible covering of the grain that protects it from the wind, cold and other elements until it sprouts. This is the portion of the grain that provides fiber.

❒ **Hull.** An indigestible papery jacket that covers grains like rice, oats, and barley.

Once a grain has been refined, only the starchy endosperm will remain. This refining process transform a carb from heaven into a carb from hell.

A Kernel of Truth

The modern milling of whole grains supplies foods that look and taste good, but lack vital nutrients and health-protecting compounds. The refining process removes the hull, the outer bran, and the inner germ layers, leaving only the starchy endosperm. Next, this starchy remainder is ground into smaller particles of refined flour. Most of the nutrients are left behind with the bran and germ. Fiber, essential oils, and vitamin E are stripped away along with antioxidants, lignan, and other healthful plant compounds. The graph below shows the nutrients that are left in refined wheat. As you can see, refined carbohydrates will not satisfy your body's nutritional needs, which will cause you to crave more carbohydrates. This means more dead calories and the extra weight that goes with it.

No matter how you slice it, whole grain breads and other whole grain products are the best choices for good health and good taste. Not surprisingly, Americans

Nutrient Content of Refined White Flour

The following graph shows the percentage of the remaining nutrients found in white flour after it has been refined.

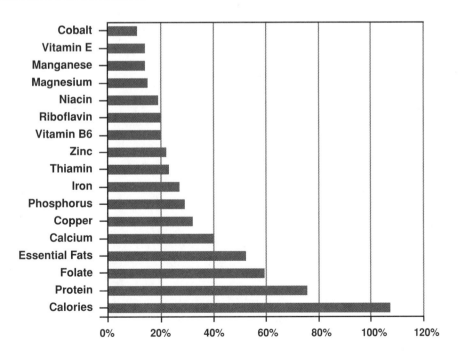

get less than 5 percent of their total food intake from whole grains. Yet, over forty medical studies have found that people who eat whole grains have up to 60-percent less incidence of stomach and colon cancer. The Nurses Health Study conducted by the Harvard Medical School followed 80,000 women for more than ten years, and discovered that those who ate two to three servings of whole grains per day lowered their incidence of heart disease by up to 40 percent. Those who ate the most whole grains had a 43-percent lowered risk for strokes. Another study conducted at the Harvard School of Public Health showed that regular consumption of whole grains lowered the risk of diabetes by 30 percent. Doesn't it make sense to incorporate whole grains into your diet?

The best news is that you don't have to give up your favorite cookies, pies, or breads to gain all of these benefits. Simply replace the white flour and other refined ingredients with unrefined carbohydrates, and you're good to go!

Chromium, Nature's Weight-Loss Mineral

Although carbs are rich sources of all the essential minerals, it is worth mentioning one of these minerals that can help you win the battle of the bulge—chromium. This important trace mineral is needed only in tiny amounts, yet it has a significant influence on blood sugar levels and weight control. Chromium helps make insulin work more efficiently, which some researchers believe can help you lose weight.

Promising research also indicates chromium can help reduce body fat and increase lean muscle mass. Whole grain wheat, rye, and corn are some of the best sources of chromium. Unfortunately, 80 percent of Americans rarely eat whole grain foods, making it difficult to receive adequate amounts of this mineral. Many scientists believe chromium deficiency may be one of the leading causes of obesity in the United States. To make matters worse, carbohydrates from hell, like white sugar and white flour, deplete the body's stores of chromium by triggering its elimination through the urine. Carbohydrates from heaven are rich sources of chromium. The foods listed in the inset on page 53 are the most concentrated dietary sources of chromium.

In addition to chromium, several other nutrients, including the mineral selenium, vitamins C and E, and a long list of disease-fighting plant compounds, are found in whole grains. It is important to recognize that many of these vital nutrients are not available in animal-based foods, which makes eating carbohydrates imperative to ensure good health. Scientists have discovered many compounds in grains and beans that restore and maintain good health. For example, soybeans have antioxidants that help protect women from estrogen-driven breast cancers.

Whole grains have plant lignans, which help prevent several different cancer types. Whole grains and beans are rich sources of fiber. Most people think of fiber as "roughage," a bulking agent to maintain regular bowel function. But it has many more benefits. Scientists have discovered that certain types of fiber can regulate blood sugar, lower cholesterol and blood pressure, and even reduce the risk of certain types of cancer.

Chromium Levels of Specific Foods

The following chromium levels, measured in micrograms (mcg), are based on a single serving (100 grams) of the following foods.

Whole Wheat Bread	42 mcg	Apple	14 mcg	Spinach	10 mcg
Whole Rye Bread	30 mcg	Parsnips	13 mcg	Carrots	9 mcg
Potatoes with skins	24 mcg	Cornmeal	12 mcg	Navy Beans	8 mcg
Green Pepper	19 mcg	Banana	10 mcg	Blueberries	5 mcg

Carbohydrates are more than just vitamins, minerals, and phytonutrients. They are whole complex foods with an assembly of nutrients that work together in concert—rather than isolated parts. Although scientists analyze the benefits of separate nutrients, we should not forget that the miraculous compounds found in carbohydrates work together as a team.

An Apple a Day . . . Really Does Keep the Doctor Away

Increasing your daily consumption of apples, along with some grapes, pears, broccoli, tomatoes, green peppers, garlic, whole grains, and beans will provide your body with the fighting power to combat more than sixty diseases, including heart disease, arthritis, and cancer, before they even get started. Food chemists have discovered thousands of compounds inside carbohydrates that act as *antioxidants*, one of nature's secret disease-fighting weapons that also serves as the body's natural line of defense against the ravages of aging. But before further explaining the role of antioxidants, I must first backtrack a bit and provide some important background information.

The basic building block of life is a cell. Every living thing, from pears to bears, is made up of cells. Left unprotected, cells can quickly deteriorate, mutate, or die.

Safeguarding cells from injury is essential for maintaining a healthy body. One of the biggest threats to our cells' well-being are harmful compounds known as *free radicals*, which are as wild and unfriendly as their name implies. Free radicals are "toxic waste"—the aftermath of many of the body's normal activities, such as converting oxygen into energy, and fighting bacteria and viruses. Stress, injury, and exposure to chemicals in the air, food, and water, also increase the presence of free radicals.

The destructive forces of free radicals create wild chain reactions that can rapidly get out of control. It is this uncontrolled activity that makes them so dangerous to living organisms. They damage cell walls, tearing them apart and eventually disabling or destroying them. Enter disease. Free radicals are a constant threat to the health and well-being of all body cells, tissues, and organs. So how does the body combat them? With antioxidants.

Picture yourself scuba diving into the microscopic world of your bloodstream. Free radicals are everywhere; they are like beams of light, wildly crashing into other beams of light, seeking to damage cells. The body's defenses are left unprotected and helpless as the free radicals attack. Cells are staggering and dying. But wait, swimming ahead is a rescue team that looks like the Navy Seals. It turns out they are the body's own armed forces—antioxidants. These special defenses quickly neutralize the free radicals and render them harmless. Antioxidants are on constant vigil, twenty-four hours a day, protecting the body from harmful free-radical reactions. They are an integral part of our body's natural defense against infection, stress, and pollution.

Our bodies make their own antioxidants, but the supply can run out, even under normal circumstances. Without this protection, we would die prematurely, so it is important to replenish our antioxidant reserves from the foods we eat. Which foods do you suppose contain the most antioxidants? If your answer is carbohydrates from heaven, give yourself a star. Food scientists have discovered that antioxidants are locked inside fresh fruits and vegetables, grains, beans, and legumes. Each type of antioxidant works best in a different part of the body, so a broad spectrum of these free-radical fighters is essential for maximum health and protection. Whole, unprocessed plant foods provide an array of antioxidant compounds that are not available in animal foods. Substituting carbohydrates with excess amounts of animal foods is a costly mistake. Doing so creates a deficiency of vital nutrients, eventually leading to disease and premature death.

Fats are one of the central free-radical targets. The brain is about 60 percent fat. In order for the brain and nervous system to protect their fat stores from free radicals, they require a high level of antioxidant nutrients. Researchers have demonstrated that animals who are fed a diet that is stripped of antioxidants quickly develop brain damage. Deposits of the harmful protein *lipofuscin* were discovered in the brains of these antioxidant-deficient animals. The buildup of lipofuscin in the brain has been linked to brain cell damage, Alzheimer's disease, and accelerated brain aging. It is quite obvious that antioxidants play a major role in protecting the integrity and function of not only the brain and nervous system, but the entire body as well.

There are two simple ways you can help your body protect itself from harmful free radicals. First, eat at least five to seven servings of fresh fruits and vegetables, and six to nine servings of whole grains, beans, and legumes every day. Second, take a multiple-vitamin-and-mineral supplement that also contains whole-food plant antioxidants. These simple measures will provide your body with plenty of ammunition to fight free radicals.

Start Roughing It!

Fiber is almost always associated with improved bowel function, but its important role in other areas of health remains somewhat of a mystery. Dietary fiber can help you lose weight; lower cholesterol and blood pressure; balance blood sugar levels; and reduce your risk for diabetes, heart disease and cancer.

The link between inadequate dietary fiber intake and disease is well established in medical literature. One of the leading world authorities on this subject is Dr. Dennis Buerkitt, M.D. For over twenty years, Dr. Buerkitt has been studying the health habits and disease patterns of populations from around the world. Through extensive documentation, he eventually formulated the *fiber theory of disease,* which basically states that low-fiber diets are the cause of many degenerative diseases. He based his theory on the rate of disease found in different world populations.

While practicing medicine in Africa, Buerkitt noticed that the natives, who worked for the British naval officers stationed there, rarely experienced the diseases that their British counterparts suffered. This prompted him to compare the high-fiber diet of the natives with the low-fiber, refined diet of the British. He specifically used the officers' wives as study subjects.

When observing stool transit time—the amount of time it takes for the food to enter the mouth and then exit the body—Buerkitt discovered that the Africans had an eighteen- to twenty-four-hour transit time, while the average time for the officers' wives was forty-eight to ninety-six hours. Buerkitt also noted that the average weight of the natives' stool was approximately sixteen ounces. The stool of the naval officers' wives' averaged five ounces. The most revealing observation of Buerkitt's work was that although the officers' wives' suffered from a long list of degenerative diseases, which are associated with a low-fiber diet (see the inset below), the native Africans were virtually free from them.

Buerkitt concluded that the factor responsible for the dramatic difference in the health of the two population groups was the amount of fiber in their diet. What is most interesting, is that when the natives adopted the diet of the naval officers' wives, they began developing the same diseases as their British counterparts. Other researchers, in different locations around the world, with no association to Buerkitt, have observed the same pattern in different cultures. Dr. Buerkitt's comprehensive work on the fiber theory of disease can be found in *Western Diseases: Their Emergence and Prevention*, a work he co-authored with Dr. Hugh Trowell, M.D.

Diseases and Conditions Linked to a Low-Fiber Diet

Scientific researchers have linked the following illnesses and health problems to a low-fiber diet.

Systemic: Diabetes, obesity, kidney stones, gall stones, gout.
Cardiovascular: High blood pressure, stroke, heart attack, varicose veins.
Other: Cavities, multiple sclerosis, thyroid conditions, skin disorders, autoimmune disorders.

Common Sense Medicine

What can we learn from Buerkitt's work? A high-fiber diet leads to shorter stool transit time and good health. A low-fiber diet leads to longer transit time, constipation, and poor health. The diet of the average American and British adult includes 10 to 12 grams of fiber per day (low-carb diets provide even less), and results in a stool transit time of approximately forty-eight to ninety-six hours. The average African, whose traditional diet includes 100 to 150 grams of fiber per day, has an eighteen- to twenty-four-hour stool transit time. Low-carb diets provide even less fiber. (See page 270 for Stool Transit Time Test.)

The American Heart Association recommends 20 to 35 grams of fiber per day (one-fourth the intake of the healthy African natives in Buerkitt's study). Some people with poor-fiber diets try to compensate by taking fiber supplements. Although these supplements may have a role in the initial treatment of some diseases, it should be emphasized that there is no substitute for the fiber that comes from whole natural foods. Studies indicate that the benefits of fiber supplements are significantly reduced when refined carbohydrates make up as little as 18 percent of the total dietary calories. It is quite clear that nature intended us to eat the whole food—the fiber along with the starch found in carbohydrates from heaven.

Just be careful when selecting high-fiber foods. For example, popcorn is a carbohydrate from heaven and makes a great-tasting high-fiber snack—unless you purchase it at the movies, where it has been transformed into a carbohydrate from hell. A tub of movie popcorn can contain as much fat as that found in five Big Macs! Theatre-style popcorn and similar brands are loaded with hydrogenated oils, which promote hardening of the arteries. Sugar-coated popcorn is just as bad, and caramel corn can contain up to 450 calories per one-cup serving. Try hot air popcorn and season it with your favorite herbs, Bragg Liquid Aminos (unfermented, liquid protein—similar to soy sauce—that contains essential and nonessential amino acids), or a light sprinkling of a 1-to-1 butter-olive oil mixture.

Good health depends as much upon good elimination as it does upon the quality of the food we consume. Although we cannot overestimate the value of getting bad things out of our bodies, we often underestimate the value of putting good things in. One common problem of a low-carb diet is constipation. Nutrient dense and fiber rich carbs from heaven, help prevent constipation, toxic bowel, and diseases associated with delayed transit time. Constipation costs Americans $725 million a year in over-the-counter laxatives, and results in 2 million yearly doctor visits. In light of the serious problems that can arise from a decreased stool transit time and constipation, anyone on a low-carb diet should be concerned.

I find it interesting that many conventional doctors claim that forty-eight to ninety-six hours is a normal stool transit time. I have consulted with patients who were advised by their doctors that having a bowel movement once every two weeks was normal for them. No wonder so many Americans are sick. Some health care providers don't understand the connection between bowel function and disease. Yet, Buerkitt's research proved that stool transit time is important to overall health. If a sluggish bowel becomes a chronic condition, health is compromised.

Considering the obvious correlation between low fiber and disease, common sense should dictate that we increase our daily fiber intake to at least 50 grams. Unfortunately, in our modern era, drugs and surgery have replaced common-sense medicine. Perhaps our health care policy makers should take the advice of nineteenth-century American humorist Henry Wheeler Shaw, who said, "A good set of bowels is worth more to a man than any quantity of brains."

The Best Sources of Fiber

Food	Quantity	Grams of Fiber
FRUIT		
Figs, dried	5	12.0
Apple, with skin	1	5.7
Pear	1	5.0
Raisins	1/2 cup	5.0
Raspberries	1/2 cup	4.2
Blackberries	1/2 cup	3.8
Dates	5	3.2
Orange	1	3.4
Prunes	5	3.0
Strawberries	1/2 cup	3.0
Kiwi fruit	1	3.0
Banana	1	2.8
Nectarine	1	2.2
Cantaloupe	1/2 melon	2.2
Blueberries	1/2 cup	2.0
VEGETABLES		
Potato, with skin	1	3.8
Sweet potato, with skin	1	3.4
Parsnips	1/2 cup	3.1
Asparagus	1 cup	2.8
Brussels sprouts	5	2.7
Broccoli	1 cup	2.6
Turnip greens, boiled	1/2 cup	2.5
Cauliflower	5 florets	2.4
Corn	1 ear	2.4
Parsley, chopped	1 cup	2.0

The Best Sources of Fiber

Food	Quantity	Grams of Fiber
VEGETABLES		
Green beans	1/2 cup	2.0
Carrot	1	1.8
Zucchini	1/2 cup	1.7
Cabbage	1 cup	1.6
Spinach	1/2 cup	0.4
BEANS & LEGUMES		
Split peas	1/2 cup	8.2
Lentils	1/2 cup	7.8
Pinto beans	1/2 cup	7.4
Kidney beans	1/2 cup	6.5
Lima beans	1/2 cup	6.5
Chick peas (garbanzo)	1/2 cup	6.2
Navy beans	1/2 cup	5.8
White beans	1/2 cup	5.7
Black-eyed peas	1/2 cup	5.5
GRAINS		
Rolled oats, dry	1/2 cup	2.0
Wild rice, cooked	1/2 cup	1.5
Millet, dry	1/2 cup	1.2
PASTA NOODLES		
Triticale, dry	1/2 cup	9.5
Quinoa, dry	1/2 cup	5.0
Whole wheat, dry	1/2 cup	4.5
NUTS		
Almonds	2 ounces	6.7

Source: USDA National Nutrient Database for Standard Reference

Nature's Appetite Suppressant

If you're trying to slim down, take advantage of fiber—a safe appetite suppressant, compliments of nature. High-fiber foods like grains and beans attract water and then swell inside the stomach, creating a sense of fullness. Consequently, the brain gets the message that hunger has been satisfied. High-fiber foods also satisfy hunger longer than refined foods, which have been stripped of their fiber.

The human digestive tract is designed to accommodate large quantities of fiber. Our ancestors ate 100 grams of fiber or more per day—a far cry from the scant 12 grams found in the diet of today's average American. But don't worry, in Chapter 13, I'll show you how to easily get 50 grams of fiber per day through my delicious American-MediterrAsian diet.

I recommend including more fiber in your diet (the Table on pages 58 and 59 offers an extensive list), but do so gradually. By adding 3 to 4 grams of fiber every few days, you can avoid any uncomfortable side effects, such as bloating and intestinal gas, which may occur with added fiber. You can also purchase digestive enzyme supplements in a health food store to help break down and assimilate beans and grains without the discomfort of gas and bloating.

Summing It Up

This chapter has provided the basics, the foundation of information on carbohydrates. It has detailed their components and nutritional value, and has shown the difference between good carbs and bad—carbs from heaven and carbs from hell. But there is a lot more to learn about this primary source of fuel for the body. The next chapter explains the role of carbohydrates in controlling blood sugar levels, which is of critical importance in avoiding a number of illnesses and health conditions, as well as controlling proper weight.

Chapter Five

Carbohydrates and Biochemical Imbalances

By now, you have a pretty good idea of what carbohydrates are. You also know the difference between the good ones and the bad. This chapter further discusses the role of carbohydrates—specifically their effect on blood sugar levels. You'll also become aware of the connection between refined carbs and behavioral disorders.

Blood Sugar Control

Carbohydrates from heaven and carbohydrates from hell are metabolized into one simple sugar called *glucose*—also known as blood sugar. Glucose is the body's main source of fuel, providing energy for the brain, muscles, and virtually every other cell in the body. Like gasoline provides fuel for automobiles, glucose provides fuel for the body. If your car runs out of gas, it will stop. If your body runs out of glucose, you will die.

The body has self-regulating "on-off" switches to keep blood sugar levels from getting too high or too low. These levels are maintained within a specific range to provide fuel for cells on a second-to-second basis. Quick shifts in either direction result in low or high blood sugar levels, which can stress cells and disrupt normal function. If blood sugar levels drop too low, the individual may become tired, irritable, or experience headaches as the cells run out of fuel. If the levels become too high over an extended period of time, diabetes can result. The high sugar levels of diabetes can damage cells, leading to infections, clogged arteries, heart disease, and even blindness.

Stable blood sugar levels are one of the most important considerations in maintaining physical and mental well-being. Most blood sugar problems are triggered by excesses of refined carbohydrates like white sugar, soda pop, candy, and refined wheat products. Refined breads, pastries, and pastas, for example, are digested and absorbed quickly—almost as quickly as white sugar. An excess of refined carbohydrates can cause blood sugar levels to shift from one extreme to another.

The amount of glucose in your blood fluctuates throughout the day. After a snack or a meal, the level automatically rises. During physical and mental activity, blood sugar is burned as fuel and the level drops. If the level drops too low between meals, the body will draw *glycogen* (sugar) from its reserves in the muscles or liver.

The body behaves differently after eating carbohydrates from heaven and those from hell. Carbs from heaven are slowly absorbed into the blood, releasing sugar slowly. By contrast, carbs from hell are absorbed quickly, releasing a surge of sugar into the bloodstream; this creates imbalance and places a burden on the body. Scientists have designed a tool called the glycemic index (page 99), which measures the rate of absorption of the sugars found in foods. It ranks foods according to how high they raise blood sugar levels. Although this dietary tool has value, it can be misleading if the person using it does not have a full understanding of its flaws and limitations. This information is detailed in Chapter 6.

Metabolism of a Carbohydrate

Let's take a closer look at how the sugar that is stored within a carbohydrate is transported into the bloodstream, and reaches its final destination inside a cell.

Once a bowl of oatmeal or a bean burrito enters the stomach, its high-fiber content (the indigestible carbohydrate) prevents it from leaving the stomach too quickly, which helps maintain a feeling a fullness. The next stop for the foodstuff is the small intestine, where the fiber unravels itself from the starch (the digestible carbohydrate). At this point, the starch pushes itself through the thick, sludge-like fiber and slowly makes its way toward the *villi*—the tiny fingerlike projections of the small intestine where absorption occurs. The slow, methodical movement of the starch delays the absorption of the sugar into the blood.

By the time the starch reaches the villi, it has been broken down into glucose and is ready to be escorted into the blood. Once the glucose enters the bloodstream, the blood sugar level rises. This, in turn, alerts the pancreas, which secretes *insulin*, a hormone that helps transport the glucose into the cells. As glucose enters the cells, some of it is used immediately as fuel, while a portion is stored in the liver and muscles as reserve fuel. Any remaining glucose is stored as fat. As the glucose is distributed throughout the body, blood sugar levels start to fall. Just in time for dinner.

Carbohydrates from hell, however, do not generate this same type of normal response. They are troublemakers because of their high-starch content and little or no fiber. Once the calorie-rich, nutrient-poor starch reaches the stomach, it is quickly carted to the small intestines—there is no fiber to delay its stay in the stomach.

Once in the intestines, without fiber to allow for gradual absorption, the starch is rapidly absorbed into the bloodstream. This causes a quick surge of glucose in the blood, which triggers a sudden elevation in blood sugar levels. The pancreas then releases a spike of insulin, which goes to work immediately. First, the insulin transports the glucose into the cells, then it mops up the excess glucose.

Excess levels of insulin may cause blood sugar levels to drop below normal, resulting in *hypoglycemia*—a state of low blood sugar. Hypoglycemia indicates the body is starving for glucose. Individuals with low blood sugar typically experience symptoms such as fatigue, irritability, "fuzziness" in the head, dizziness, headache, and/or a craving for carbohydrates. Millions of Americans experience one or more of these common symptoms every day. And carbohydrates from hell are often the cause; they are deficient in the fiber, vitamins, and minerals that are vital for maintaining stable blood sugar levels. The charts on page 70 further illustrate the different blood sugar responses caused by carbohydrates from heaven and those from hell.

Insulin Resistance

Eating too many refined carbohydrates year after year can trigger *insulin resistance*—a debilitating condition in which cells become less responsive to insulin. To put it simply, insulin knocks at the door of the cells, requesting permission to enter with a supply of glucose; but many of the cells can't hear its voice. Consequently, the insulin remains on the outside of the cells looking in. To compensate, more insulin is produced in an attempt to get the attention of those cells that are unable to hear it. As a result, insulin levels remain chronically high. Blood sugar levels also remain high because the insulin is unable to deliver it into the cells. At that point, insulin resistance can spiral into type II diabetes, also known as noninsulin dependent diabetes. About 90 percent of all diabetics have this acquired form of the disease. In the Harvard Nurses Study of 80,000 women, those who ate the most refined carbohydrates and the least amount of whole grains, had a two-and-a-half time greater risk of developing type II diabetes.

Although insulin resistance is a complex condition, basically, it means that insulin has a reduced ability to move glucose into the cells. Because of this, the body becomes starved for energy, and results in a number of possible side effects, including fatigue, a craving for sweets, sleep problems, mood swings, muscle aches and pains, irritable bowel syndrome, and many other symptoms. Furthermore, a number of scientists believe that chronically high insulin levels stimulate the production of fat. This is why people who are insulin resistant may have a difficult time losing weight.

It is estimated that insulin resistance affects 70 to 80 million people, or one out of every four Americans. About 25 percent of those affected do not have any symptoms. They do, however, have a high risk of developing several of the problems associated with this syndrome. Left unresolved, insulin resistance can lead to a more serious condition known as *Syndrome X*, which may result in obesity, diabetes, high blood pressure, heart disease, polycystic ovaries, and possibly even cancer. (More details of this condition are presented in Chapter 7.)

If you suspect that you may have insulin resistance, what should you do? I suggest first talking to your doctor, who, with your cooperation, should be able to help improve your body's ability to use insulin more efficiently. But be sure to take a proactive role. Eliminate or radically reduce your intake of carbohydrates from hell. In addition, avoid hydrogenated fats, such as margarine and refined vegetable oils, and minimize your consumption of foods that are high in saturated fat, like beef, pork, and chicken. These are all risk factors for insulin resistance. Follow the eating strategy outlined in the American-MediterrAsian diet presented in Chapter 13. As you will see, this diet can be modified to meet your personal tastes.

What's important to remember is that you don't have to give up your favorite carbohydrate foods to help restore the action of insulin. Simply substitute the refined ingredients in your favorite recipes with unrefined carbohydrates from heaven. To experience the variety and extraordinary tastes of unrefined carbohydrate foods, be sure to try some of the recipes presented in Chapter 14.

The High Complex-Fiber (HCF) Diet

One of the most effective diets for controlling blood sugar levels and minimizing insulin resistance is the high complex-fiber (HCF) diet, which is effective for treating both insulin-dependent (type I) and noninsulin-dependent (type II) diabetics. Although many alternative-health doctors have used variations of the HCF diet for decades, James Anderson M.D., of the University of Kentucky Medical School, popularized it. Dr. Anderson's research with the HCF diet has received a great deal of attention in prestigious medical journals. One study found that type I insulin-dependent diabetics who had been following the diet recommended by the American Diabetic Association (ADA), and then switched to the HCF diet, were able to significantly reduce their need for insulin. Most interestingly, when these individuals reintroduced the ADA diet, their need for insulin reverted back to the original levels.

The HCF diet relies on a whopping 75 percent of unrefined carbohydrates from whole grains, beans, legumes, and root vegetables. Along with this, Dr. Anderson also restricts refined carbohydrates and saturated fat. The total caloric intake from fat is anywhere from 10 to 25 percent, and the total protein is from 15 to 25 percent. Once the individual is stabilized, Dr. Anderson modifies the intake of these foods.

The HCF diet is considered one of the most effective diets for diabetics, and its benefits are well documented in scientific literature. It increases the body's sensitivity to insulin, reduces blood sugar levels, and increases HDL cholesterol (the "good" cholesterol). The HCF diet also decreases total cholesterol and triglyceride levels, and stimulates progressive weight loss.

A "Pair-of-Docs" and a "Paradox" on Low-Carb Diets

Low-carb diet doctors often refer to the increased incidence of insulin resistance, and conventional medicine's failure to stop the growing cases of diabetes and heart disease that are associated with it. They believe that limiting carbohydrates and increasing the intake of fat will reverse these problems. Dr. Robert Atkins, for instance, claimed that his low-carb, high-protein diet could solve the problems associated with insulin resistance. His personal goal was to win the battle against diabetes and heart disease. Here is what Dr. Anderson had to say in response to Dr. Atkins' claims. "People lose weight, at least in the short term. But this is absolutely the worst diet you can imagine for long-term obesity, heart disease, and some forms of cancer. If you wanted to find one diet to ruin your health, you couldn't find one worse than Atkins. We have 18 million diabetics in this country, 50 million people with high blood pressure. They can have kidney problems, and high-protein intake will bring them on faster. The diet is thrombogenic, meaning that fat will tend to form lipid particles in your blood after meals, which could lead to blood clots, meaning heart attack or stroke. We worry about this, because many of the people who love these diets are men age forty to fifty, who like their meat. They may be five years from their first heart attack. This couldn't be worse for them. Did you know that for 50 percent of men who die from heart attacks, the fatal attack is the first symptom? They will never know what this diet is doing to them."

Start Moving to Improve Insulin Resistance

One of the many benefits of exercise is that it helps make insulin-resistant cells become more responsive when insulin comes knocking at the door. A combination of aerobic and weight-training exercises can significantly increase cell sensitivity to insulin. Research studies indicate that a brisk daily walk can vastly improve the body's ability to handle blood sugar more efficiently. According to Dr. Ralph S. Paffenberger, M.D.,

Ph.D., and professor emeritus of epidemiology at Stanford School of Medicine, "The risk of type II diabetes is reduced by 25 percent, and the risk of heart disease by 50 percent among people who are moderately active, compared to those who are sedentary."

Dr. Jean-Pierre Despres, Ph.D., director of the Lipid Research Center at Laval University Hospital in Quebec, Canada, puts the same message another way. He says, "Exercise is probably the best medication on the market to treat insulin resistance syndrome. Our studies show that low intensity, prolonged exercise—such as a daily brisk walk of forty-five minutes to an hour—will substantially reduce insulin levels, and reduce apo-B (sub fractions of cholesterol) concentrations, thus reducing the risk of both diabetes and heart disease."

Vitamins to the Rescue

Scientists have found that vitamin and mineral supplements can help make insulin work more effectively, make tissues more sensitive to insulin, and stabilize blood sugars. A good multiple vitamin with at least 500 milligrams (mg) of vitamin C, and 400 International Units (IU) of vitamin E will provide a foundation for effective sugar control. The following supplements are key nutrients in helping to reverse the symptoms of insulin resistance.

❒ **Multiple vitamin-and-mineral formula with extra antioxidants**
Provides a good foundational supplement.

❒ **Chromium pincolonate** (200 mcg/1x per day)
Improves glucose tolerance, decreases fasting glucose levels, helps insulin work more efficiently. Decreases body fat and increases lean muscle mass.

❒ **Omega-3 fatty acids** (1,000 to 3,000 mg per day)
Decreases risk of heart disease. A deficiency causes increased insulin resistance and subsequent diabetes.

❒ **Guar gum or pectin** (5 grams/3x per day)
Helps to slow down the absorption of sugar.

❒ **Vitamin C** (500 mg/2x per day)
Decreases fasting insulin levels, LDL cholesterol levels (the "bad" cholesterol), and total cholesterol levels above 200.

❒ **Fenugreek seeds** (25 mg/1x per day)
Reduces fasting blood sugar levels, and increases cell sensitivity to insulin.

Carbohydrates and Behavioral Disorders

Food—carbohydrates, protein, and fat—provides vitamins, minerals, and phyto-chemicals to build hormones, enzymes, and bone. It also provides fuel for energy and cell repair, and for running the immune system. But food is so much more than just a bundle of raw elements. It is a central part of our family traditions, celebrations, special events, and entertainment. And let's be honest, carbohydrates have always played a major role in our enjoyment of food. Remember as a youngster, the excitement of seeing your birthday cake aglow with candles as friends and family sang to you, or the warm feeling you received from a bowl of mom's hot oatmeal cereal before heading off to school? What about the fond memory of family picnics with ears of roasted corn on the cob, potato and macaroni salad, baked beans, and homemade apple pie? Carbohydrates are much more than mere calories that provide energy to burn. They are foods that also affect our moods and behavior.

Most health experts agree that food affects behavior. According to Dr. Simon N. Young, professor in the Department of Psychiatry at McGill University, "No one doubts that food can influence mood and behavior, but the mechanisms by which this happens are not fully understood." Several good theories of how food alters mood already exist. Let's explore a few of these theories that focus on the role of carbs from heaven and carbs from hell.

Mind-Body Connection

We can live without water for days, but our brains cannot survive without glucose and oxygen for more than minutes. Proper nutrition is critical for brain function, health, and survival. It is important to remember that all nutrients known to man are essential for optimal brain function. A deficiency of just one nutrient can cause a problem; however, certain nutrients are more critical than others.

All of the B vitamins, the entire complex, are probably the most highly regarded nutrients for optimal functioning of the brain and nervous system. Several other all-star nutrients, including the minerals calcium, magnesium, iron, and zinc; the amino acids tryptophan, tyrosine, and taurine; and omega-3 and omega-6 essential fatty acids, also play an important role. All of these nutrients are found in carbohydrates from heaven; in carbohydrates from hell, many are missing or severely deficient.

Throughout the life cycle, vitamin and mineral levels play a vital role in the brain and nervous system—particularly in the aging process. Several decades of research have demonstrated this. For instance, the 1980's research of Derick Lonsdale, M.D., and Dr. Raymond Shamberger noted that individuals with low levels of B vitamins exhibited a wide variety of neurological symptoms: depression, sleep disturbances, personality changes, repeated episodes of bad dreams, fatigue, and abdominal and chest pains. Once the nutrient deficiencies were corrected, the symptoms disappeared.

In another study, researchers at the United States Department of Agriculture tested the mental performance of individuals who were under stress. They discovered that even minor vitamin or mineral deficiencies resulted in significant changes in brain chemistry and mental capacity. Researchers have shown that nutrition controls the release of brain chemicals that alter the mind's memory, moods, and behaviors.

Food, Mood, and Behavior

A growing body of research suggests foods can alter our brain chemistry the same way antidepressants and mind-altering drugs do. Two mechanisms by which foods affect brain chemistry are food allergies and blood sugar fluctuations.

Several research studies have demonstrated a high incidence of food allergies in individuals with clinical depression. Research scientists at Harvard Medical School of Psychiatry found that over 70 percent of the patients in their study with depression had a history of allergies.

Dr. James Braly, a medical doctor and a leading authority on food allergies and sensitivities states, "Whether we look at depression, anxiety, or behavioral disturbance, such psychiatric symptoms are often eliminated by the simple removal of gluten (wheat, barley, rye, oats) from the diet." Using the effective ELISA (enzyme-linked immunosorbent assay) food allergy blood test, Dr. Braly has supervised tests on tens of thousands of patients. A significant percentage of these patients has shown a dramatic improvement in depression, mood swings, aggression, hyperactivity, and irritability once the offending foods were eliminated. I have found similar results with thousands of my own patients.

Although food allergies can alter brain chemistry, the exact mechanisms that trigger these biochemical changes are not clearly understood. However, since the identification and elimination of hidden food allergies can't cause any harm, I believe it is worthwhile to explore these allergies as a potential cause for any type of behavioral disorder.

Lick the Sugar Habit, Before You
Start Singing the Sugar Blues

"Ev'rbody's singing the Sugar Blues. . . . I'm so unhappy, I feel so bad I could lay me down and die. You can say what you choose, but I'm confused. I've got the sweet, sweet, Sugar Blues. More Sugar! I've got the sweet, sweet Sugar Blues."

Back in the 1920s, sugar inspired the blues, but today, Americans eat so much sugar they are living the blues. The average American consumes approximately 150 pounds of sugar a year, about a half cup per day. On top of that, they also eat an inordinate amount of other sweeteners, including corn syrup, high fructose corn syrup, dextrose, glucose, and maltose, to name just a few. It's hard to believe, but many doctors, dieticians, and government organizations insist that sugar is safe, claiming the dangers are myths.

In 1986, the Food and Drug Administration (FDA) reported that excess sugar in the diet could have serious health consequences. The report was based on scientific studies published in medical journals, not on the FDA's own research. The report stated that overconsumption of sugar, specifically more than 25 to 50 percent of total daily calorie intake, could result in one or more serious health risks, including heart disease, diabetes, low blood sugar, behavioral problems, depletion of calcium and other minerals, and gallstones. The report went on to assure Americans not to be concerned with these risks, since sugar made up less than 25 percent of the average American diet. However, according to the government's National Research Council 1989 report entitled, "Diet and Health: implications for reducing chronic disease risk," more than 30 percent of the total daily calorie intake of the average American is from refined sugars. The percent of sugar in the American diet has certainly increased since the publication of this nearly two-decades old report. This is a disturbing fact, particularly in light of the FDA report. Has your doctor ever alerted you to these important medical findings?

The Sour Side of Sugar

In the 1970s, there were many heated discussions on the harmful effects of sugar. The book *Sugar Blues* by William Duffy warned of these dangers, but the claims were received by the medical community with a great deal of skepticism. Prestigious medical journals like *The New England Journal of Medicine* tried to discourage the public's association between sugar and illness. Despite any efforts to ignore the evidence of the sugar-illness connection, plenty of new evidence has emerged.

In the 1970s, *hypoglycemia* (low blood sugar) was the buzzword for a condition linked to too much sugar. Today, new terms like reactive hypoglycemia, insulin resistance, and Syndrome X are used to describe the same old problem—the sugar blues. Hypoglycemia can cause a wide range of symptoms, often diagnosed as psychosomatic, or "all in the head."

Normally, blood sugar levels stay within a narrow range, but if a diet is low in fiber and loaded with refined carbohydrates (the standard American diet), sugar levels will fluctuate, high and low. As discussed earlier in this chapter, a meal with carbs from hell will cause a rapid spike in blood sugar levels, which signals the pancreas to release insulin into the blood. In the case of hypoglycemia, unlike insulin resistance, the cells respond quickly to the excess insulin, which causes blood sugar levels to plummet. The charts below compare a normal blood sugar response to the response in the case of hypoglycemia.

During this downward spiral, the brain is shortchanged of its glucose supply, which can trigger some very bizarre symptoms. If the blood sugar drops low enough, brain function may become impaired. A partial list of possible symptoms includes anxiety, depression, fatigue, headache, heart palpitations, inability to concentrate, nervousness, perspiration, and shakiness.

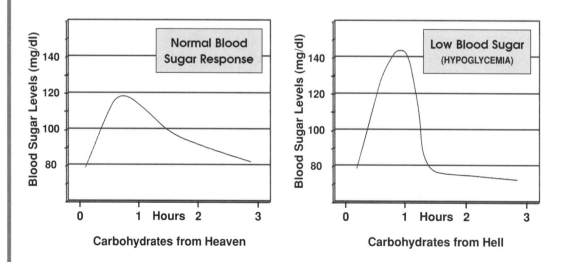

Blood Sugar Response for Carbohydrates

Normal Blood Sugar Response

Blood Sugar Levels (mg/dl)

Carbohydrates from Heaven

Low Blood Sugar (HYPOGLYCEMIA)

Blood Sugar Levels (mg/dl)

Carbohydrates from Hell

Most doctors don't pay attention to blood sugar problems—except in cases of those with diabetes. If you are experiencing one or more of the symptoms just mentioned and you suspect low blood sugar may be the cause, discuss this concern with your doctor. Ask to take a six-hour glucose tolerance test, which is designed to indicate if your blood sugar is normal. Along with this test, it is also important to have your insulin level checked. This additional insulin reading is important because the glucose test alone may provide a "false negative" result. This means that even if this test indicates your blood sugar levels are normal, you may still have hypoglycemia. About 66 percent of people with symptoms of hypoglycemia have an abnormal amount of insulin in the blood, but show normal blood sugar levels during the six-hour test period. Elevated insulin levels can cause an abrupt drop in blood sugar and result in symptoms of hypoglycemia. So be sure to have your insulin level checked along with the glucose tolerance test.

Unstable sugar levels affect the ability of tissues in the body to uptake sugar. The important thing to remember is that these abnormal levels can be stabilized by replacing carbs from hell with carbs from heaven, along with managing stress and exercising. Taking vitamin supplements is another way to help stabilize diabetes and low blood sugar. Recommended supplements are listed in the inset "Vitamins to the Rescue" on page 66.

Carbs from Hell Stress the Adrenal Glands

The adrenal glands, which produce several hormones that are essential to good health, are located directly above the kidneys. The hormones they produce help decrease inflammation, increase the body's resistance to stress, and regulate blood sugar levels and other vital body functions.

A healthy body responds to stress by increasing the production of adrenal gland hormones—commonly known as an "adrenaline rush." To further explain, if a tiger, or more likely a boss who acts like one, confronts you, your brain will signal your adrenal glands to secrete stress hormones, which will elevate your heart rate, raise your blood pressure, increase your sugar level, and alter your energy output. This sudden biochemical change is preparing the body for imminent danger. Known as the "fight or flight" response, this automatic reaction enables the body to either thwart the enemy—or quickly retreat. The mobilization of this self-defense system is an attempt to keep the body safe from harm.

In the past, humans were occasionally confronted by lions and tigers and bears (Oh my!). Today, most people never find themselves faced with this type of stressful situation; however, modern civilization has created other stressors that can be even more dangerous to our well-being. Today's everyday world is filled with a host of modern "tigers"—demanding employers, unreasonable landlords, over-programmed family schedules, rising costs, threats of terrorism, and diets that include too much sugar and carbs from hell. These modern "tigers" stretch us to our emotional and physical limits, and, over time, the unmanaged stress of modern life can exhaust the adrenal glands. The victim of adrenal exhaustion is not only susceptible to chronic fatigue, hypoglycemia, and depression, but also to a host of other problems like allergies, candidiasis (yeast overgrowth), and chronic pain.

Remember, the adrenal glands also aid the body when blood sugar levels drop. They secrete hormones to help raise the levels back to normal. However, if this process is repeated day in and day out, year after year, the adrenal glands become tired and depleted. The constant spiking and crashing of blood sugar levels caused by stress and refined-carbohydrate diets can lead to adrenal exhaustion. Those who suffer from this condition may experience symptoms that include nervousness, irritability, shakiness, exhaustion, depression, dizziness, and chronic fatigue. They tend to go through the ceiling at the drop of a pin. Cooperate with your body to prevent or repair adrenal exhaustion. Eat carbs from heaven and follow the stress-reduction principles in Part 3.

Criminal Behavior and Low Blood Sugar

In the late 1970s, I had the opportunity to hear a juvenile parole officer present a lecture on the adverse affects of sugar and refined carbohydrates on juvenile behavior. That's when I first began to observe these harmful effects in the behavior of many of my patients. I noticed that after removing carbs from hell from the diets of both young and older patients' alike, their moods and behaviors improved significantly. Unfortunately, most physicians pay little attention to the effects these carbohydrates have on behavior, relying instead on drugs.

Research studies involving violent and impulsive criminals, as well as psychiatric patients, indicate a strong connection between blood sugar levels and antisocial and aggressive behavior. Several large studies involving over 6,000 inmates from over ten correctional institutions, showed marked behavioral improvement after a reduction in their refined-carbohydrate intake.

One study involving male juveniles took place over a two-year period. A group of 174 participants was put on a sugar-restricted diet, while the remaining 102 subjects were given a controlled diet that contained the same amount of refined carbohydrates they were accustomed to. All of the subjects believed they were on a special diet. The results were dramatic. The group on the restricted sugar diet showed a marked 45-percent overall reduction in antisocial behavior. There was an 83-percent reduction in the number of assaults, 77-percent reduction in thefts, 65-percent reduction in horseplay, and a 55-percent reduction in refusal to take orders. Interestingly, the antisocial behavior changed most dramatically in the juveniles who were incarcerated for aggravated assault, robbery, rape, child molestation, arson, auto theft, vandalism, or the possession of a deadly weapon.

In an even more dramatic and larger study, 3,999 juvenile males were observed over a two-year time frame. One group was given fruit juice instead of soda pop, and popcorn or another whole grain snack instead of candy. Although those in the control group thought they were getting healthy replacement snacks, they were actually getting their normal high-sugar snacks. Those on the sugar-restricted snacks showed a most impressive behavioral improvement—100-percent reduction in suicide attempts, 75-percent reduction in the need for restraint to prevent self-inflicted harm, 42-percent reduction in disruptive behavior, and a 25-percent reduction in assaults.

Hyperactivity: Ritalin Deficiency or Sugar Overload?

The conventional medical community denies any connection between refined carbohydrates and hyperactivity. Surprisingly, there have been no medical studies to prove this connection. If, however, you ask a mother if she thinks there is a link between sugar and her child's hyperactive behavior, you'll get a much different assessment. Furthermore, if you tell her that no studies have been conducted to scientifically prove this connection, she's likely to react by saying, "You've got to be kidding me!"

Experts estimate that over 17 million children in this country have some sort of behavioral disorder. The most common of these conditions is *attention deficit disorder* (ADD). Children who are diagnosed with ADD have short attention spans; typically, they are easily distracted, impulsive, and/or hyperactive. The most common medication for treating this condition is Ritalin (methylphenidate), which decreases hyperactivity and increases attention.

The question is, are these children suffering from a Ritalin deficiency, or are they simply getting too many refined carbohydrates? The average child eats about one cup of refined sugar per day. Do you suppose there is any connection between that much sugar and hyperactivity? Over 90 percent of the Ritalin prescribed worldwide is for use in the United States. Currently, it is prescribed for more than 3 million of the country's children! The growing list of side effects caused by Ritalin includes weight loss, headaches, abdominal pain, and insomnia. Increasing numbers of concerned parents are searching for alternative treatments.

Candy bars and other sugar-sweetened snacks are favorites among children. Most kids would rather have a Snickers bar, a can of soda pop, or a chocolate Ho-Ho rather than a juicy red apple or a succulent strawberry. Isn't it ironic that we allow our children to eat these denatured, artificial foods, and then worry about the dangers of Ritalin? We need to at least acknowledge that our children's learning disorders may stem from an artificial sweet tooth. Eliminating junk carbs won't

Autism, Sugar, and Food Allergies

After David was diagnosed with autism, his mother enrolled him in a special education program. The teachers found it very difficult to work with David, because he was uncooperative, could not concentrate, and had difficulty comprehending the simplest of schoolroom tasks. For several years, David's mother went along with the conventional medical treatment for her son's condition; however, she kept searching for the cause of his problem. She believed there was hope for her son.

When David first entered my office at the age of seven, he was withdrawn, anxious, and loud. He was unable to sit for more than a few seconds without picking up objects in my office. His mother was patient and very hopeful. I suggested that we modify David's diet by removing all refined carbohydrates, red meat, and dairy products. I ordered the ELISA allergy blood test to identify any hidden foods that he may have been reacting to. I prescribed several nutrients, including flaxseed oil, black currant seed oil, and fish oils.

After following his allergy-free diet for the next several months, David's behavior changed dramatically. According to his teachers, he showed a remarkable improvement in concentration and school performance. He was also able to interact with others without aggression. Within six months, there was also a big difference in his grades. Today, after five years on the American-MediterrAsian diet and lifestyle (presented in Part 4), David behaves like a normal child and has a bright future.

cause the harm associated with Ritalin, and it might even prevent our children from climbing the walls.

Alternative health care providers typically limit a child's intake of refined carbohydrates. Many report remarkable improvements in behavior once they have been removed from the diet. I always tell my patients they have nothing to lose by simply eliminating or severely restricting carbohydrates from hell—and they might even be surprised by the positive results.

It is very important to understand that behavioral problems can be caused by multiple factors, making it difficult to pinpoint any one particular cause. Scientific research suggests that environmental toxins, genetics, nutrient deficiencies, and hidden food allergies, as well as excesses of refined carbohydrates, food colorings, and chemical additives may cause brain chemical imbalances. You and your physician must consider all of these factors when addressing behavioral disorders.

Summing It Up

The difference between the effects of carbs from heaven and those from hell on the body are remarkable. Nutrient-rich unrefined carbohydrates—loaded with fiber, vitamins, and minerals—are absorbed into the bloodstream very slowly, helping maintain stable blood sugar levels. On the other hand, refined, nutrient-deficient carbs from hell are absorbed quickly, releasing a surge of sugar into the bloodstream. This, in turn, triggers a spike of insulin. Excess insulin levels can result in a number of illnesses and health conditions. In addition to these biochemical balances and imbalances, carbs from heaven and hell each play significant roles in maintaining proper weight. The next chapter details how.

Chapter Six

"Battle of the Bulge"
Carbs from Heaven versus
Carbs from Hell

A man who got tired of following a low-carb diet decided he was going to eat a donut. But he wanted to be sure that it was God's will that he do it. So he prayed, "Dear Lord, if it's Your will that I eat this donut, I pray that when I go shopping today, you'll give me a sign and provide me with a parking spot right in front of the donut shop." Well, praise God, after circling around that parking lot thirteen times, there it was, a parking spot right smack in front of the donut shop.

Anyone trying to lose weight has plenty of company. Over 25 million Americans are currently on a weight-loss diet. Government surveys reveal that on any given day of the week, 44 percent of women and 29 percent of men are trying to lose weight. Most of them dream about donuts, bagels with cream cheese, and pizza. But surprisingly, for a growing number of dieters these days, it's not the fat that goes along with these favorite foods that they're worried about—it's the carbohydrates. This new breed of dieter believes that in order to shed those unwanted pounds, carbohydrates gotta' go. These folks are determined to push carbohydrates back to the Ice Age and fast forward the sausage and bacon—the new millennium health foods. But in their enthusiasm to lose weight, these dieters have forgotten an important history lesson—during the Ice Age, people lived only into their mid twenties.

Somehow, best-selling authors like Dr. Arthur Agatston (*The South Beach Diet*), Dr. Robert Atkins (*Dr. Atkins' Diet Revolution* and *New Diet Revolution*), Dr. Barry Sears (*The Zone*), and others have convinced millions of Americans that certain carbs are as bad as the worm inside the apple. Low-carb diet doctors' biggest gripe against carbohydrates involves the hormone insulin, which, they claim, is released into the bloodstream only when we eat carbs. Are these "carbophobic" doctors right? They also believe excess insulin circulating in the blood is linked to obesity and a host of other health problems. Do elevated insulin levels trigger obesity, high blood sugar, high cholesterol, and high blood pressure? Or is obesity the cause of elevated insulin levels and the symptoms that tag along with it? The debate rages on, and carbs are in the center ring; but, you may lose the fight to keep the weight off (or even worse, lose your health) unless you get all of the facts.

As you will see, carbs are not the only food group that raises insulin levels, and some carbs raise insulin more than others. Low-carb diet doctors ignore the fact that this country's expanding waistline is more than just a carb problem. Real carbs like whole oats, whole wheat, and potatoes with skin, along with a low saturated-fat diet can help you lose weight and lower blood sugar levels, blood pressure, and cholesterol levels. But before discussing the role of carbs in the "battle of the bulge," it's important to address another important factor—food allergies.

When Good Carbs Raise Hell

Carbs from heaven contribute to good health, unless you are allergic to them. Then, even good carbs can become your worst enemy. They can raise hell inside your body and cause a host of health problems—including the extra weight you're carrying around. As you will see, symptoms of food allergies often go far beyond wheezing, sneezing, and itching.

Gluten Sensitivity

Millions of people have undiagnosed food sensitivities or *hidden food allergies*. One of the most serious of these is the potentially life-threatening sensitivity to gluten, the protein found in wheat, barley, oats, and rye. Over 2 million people have been diagnosed with this potentially life-threatening sensitivity. Even small amounts (micrograms) of gluten can cause serious health problems. Stomach pain, bloating, and diarrhea are the most common symptoms, although muscle cramps, bone and/or joint pain, numbness and tingling in the extremities, weight loss or gain, rashes, depression, menstrual problems, anemia, and a long list of others can result.

It is not unusual for individuals with gluten sensitivity to be chronically ill and treated with medications for years with little or no relief. The condition, known as *celiac disease*, could lead to osteoporosis, miscarriage, seizures, and even cancer. Many people with celiac disease go undiagnosed for years. According to the

Celiac Foundation, 1 out of of every 130 people has the condition, but, on average, it takes ten years for the disease to be diagnosed. Only 1 in 5,000 people are diagnosed with celiac disease—97 percent of those who have it are misdiagnosed. Health experts estimate that as many as 30 million Americans are either sensitive to or allergic to gluten.

Leaky Gut Syndrome

Allergies and sensitivities to carbs and other foods have not always been such a widespread problem. Our twenty-first century lifestyle has accelerated the incidence of these conditions to epidemic proportions. Fast foods, poor nutrition, unmanaged stress, medications, alcohol, and environmental chemicals have set the stage for *leaky gut syndrome*—a major cause of hidden food allergies.

Under normal circumstances, during digestion and absorption of food, the lining of the small intestine allows nutrients to pass through it and enter the blood. However, if the lining of the intestines becomes irritated, inflamed, and damaged, it can develop pinhole tears and a "leaky gut." The leaky gut allows larger particles of food to enter the blood, triggering the immune system, which perceives them as foreign invaders, just like bacteria. Next, the immune system sounds an alarm and releases antibodies and inflammatory chemicals into the blood—as a full-blown allergic reaction gets underway. Inflammation, cell damage, and unwanted pounds can result. And this chain of biological events can trigger symptoms in any part of the body. Left untreated, symptoms can turn into chronic problems, including disease.

Delayed Food Allergies
Disease in Disguise

Mainstream physicians believe food allergies affect only 2 to 5 percent of the population, mostly children. Furthermore, allergy specialists normally diagnose and treat *immediate-onset allergic reactions,* which usually occur within the first half hour, but no more than three hours, after exposure to the offending substance. Allergists tend to focus on environmental substances like dust and mold, which usually trigger symptoms that are common and predictable—itching, rashes, hives, and breathing difficulty. Patients are normally evaluated with a skin scratch test. During this test, the doctor pricks the skin with a tiny amount of the suspected offending substance, and then sees if it causes a raised patch of skin—the sign of an immediate allergic reaction.

A more common, yet less recognized type of allergy is the *delayed food allergy,* also known as *IgG mediated allergy.* Its symptoms are not as predictable as immediate allergic reactions, because they can occur anywhere from three to seventy-two hours after exposure to the offending food. Consequently, if you eat the offending food for lunch today, you could have a reaction to it nine meals later. It is almost impossible for the average person with delayed food allergies to detect which foods are causing their symptoms because the cause and effect can be far apart, possibly separated by several meals.

Delayed food allergies can affect any tissue, organ, or system in the body. James Braly, M.D., author of *Dr. Braly's Food Allergy and Nutrition Revolution,* notes that according to documented medical evidence, there are over 150 symptoms and 100 different diseases that have been linked to hidden food allergies. (See the listing of common symptoms below.) According to Theron Randolph, M.D., one of the nation's leading food allergists, "Food allergies are one of America's most commonly undiagnosed medical conditions." He believes that up to 75 percent of all doctor visits are linked to hidden food allergies. Are your symptoms and inability to lose weight linked to hidden food allergies? Is it possible that your doctor has misdiagnosed your problem?

Common Symptoms Associated with Hidden Food Allergies

If you suffer from one or more of the following health problems, you may have a hidden food allergy. For a more comprehensive evaluation, fill out the questionnaire found on pages 82 and 83.

- Cramps, bloating, gas, heartburn
- Constipation, diarrhea, irritable bowel syndrome (IBS)
- Inflammatory bowel diseases (Crohn's disease, ulcerative colitis, etc.)
- Ear infections
- Bed-wetting
- Mood swings, depression, anxiety
- Watery, itchy eyes; blurred vision

- Dark circles or puffiness under the eyes
- Fatigue, frequent illness
- Headaches, migraines
- Insomnia
- Irregular or rapid heartbeat
- High blood pressure, chest pain
- Asthma, chronic cough, congestion
- Recurring lung infections
- Recurring urinary tract infections

- Hyperactivity, autism, attention deficit disorder (ADD)
- Poor concentration or memory
- Canker sores
- Frequent sore throat, swollen tonsils
- Muscle and joint pains, arthritis
- Postnasal drip

- Chronic sinus congestion, infection
- Diabetes, hypoglycemia
- Acne, hives, rash, itchy skin
- Excessive weight gain, binge eating, water retention
- PMS, infertility, prostatitis
- Autoimmune disorders (psoriasis, rheumatoid arthritis, lupus, etc.)

Phases of Hidden Food Allergies

In the 1930s, research scientist Dr. Hans Selye focused his efforts on proving that stress can weaken the body and eventually cause illness. He called his theory *biological stress syndrome*. According to Dr. Selye, stress is defined as any external stimulus that triggers a negative or positive response inside the body. In his book *Stress without Distress,* Dr. Selye describes the body's progressive reaction to stress in three phases—the acute-reaction (*alarm*) phase, the chronic (*adaptive*) phase, and the degenerative (*exhaustive*) phase. This three-phase theory of the body's negative reaction to stress can be used as a model for describing the body's reaction to the stress caused by hidden food allergies.

1. Alarm Phase. *When a harmful external stimulus (bacteria, cold air, allergic food) irritates the body, the body goes into an "alarm" or "reactive" phase.*

Suppose that after six months of breastfeeding, an infant is given a food that contains the common grain wheat. Although normally whole wheat is a carbohydrate from heaven, introducing it to any infant too early, can place stress on the baby's delicate digestive tract. The wheat quickly becomes a carb from hell. The baby's body perceives the wheat as a foreign invader, just like bacteria or a virus. In an attempt to defend itself, the body triggers an alarm (an acute reaction). During this phase, the body's immune system mobilizes its forces against the wheat. The reaction to the poorly digested food causes the baby's body to respond with symptoms such as diarrhea, diaper rash, or colic.

Even a baby who is exclusively breastfed may have this same type of allergic response. In such a case, it is the mother's food allergy and the subsequent antibodies that cross over in the breast milk that trigger the baby's symptoms.

Do You Have Hidden Food Allergies?

There are many symptoms commonly associated with hidden food allergies. Use this questionnaire to rate your symptoms according to how have felt over the last thirty days. (Answer questions as if you were taking no medications.) A total of 50 points or higher strongly suggests that your symptoms, including weight gain, are related to hidden food allergies, and the ELISA blood test (page 87) is recommended.

Symptom Rating Scale

0 = never   **1** = occasional mild symptoms   **2** = occasional severe symptoms
3 = frequent mild symptoms   **4** = frequent severe symptoms

General Well-Being
____ Restlessness
____ Fatigue, malaise
____ Stuttering
____ "Sick all over" feeling
____ Poor physical condition
____ **Total**

Digestive System
____ Indigestion
____ Heartburn
____ Diarrhea
____ Bloating
____ Constipation
____ Nausea and vomiting
____ Abdominal pain or cramps
____ Blood and/or mucus in stools
____ **Total**

Eyes
____ Eyes feel tired
____ Watery, red, or itchy eyes
____ Dark circles under eyes
____ Bags under eyes
____ Blurred vision
____ **Total**

Ears
____ Earaches
____ Ringing in the ears
____ Excessive wax
____ Hearing loss
____ Itchy or red ears
____ Recurrent ear infections
____ **Total**

Mouth and Throat
____ Canker sores
____ Chronic cough
____ Sore throat
____ Post nasal drip
____ Swollen, discolored tongue
____ **Total**

Lungs
____ Asthma
____ Shortness of breath
____ Chronic cough
____ Difficulty breathing
____ Lung congestion
____ Recurrent bronchitis
____ Recurrent lung infections
____ **Total**

Nose

____ Hay fever

____ Nasal congestion

____ Excessive sneezing

____ Recurrent sinus infections

____ **Total**

Head

____ Dizziness

____ Insomnia

____ Faintness

____ Facial flushing

____ Headaches, migraines

____ **Total**

Skin/hair

____ Acne

____ Hair loss

____ Hives, rash

____ Itchy, dry skin

____ **Total**

Heart

____ Chest pain

____ Rapid heartbeat

____ High blood pressure

____ Irregular or skipped beats

____ **Total**

Mind

____ Dyslexic

____ Poor memory

____ Attention deficit

____ Hyperactivity

____ Poor concentration

____ Confusion, fuzzy thinking

____ **Total**

Emotions

____ Mood swings

____ Depression, cry easily

____ Frustrated, irritable

____ Aggressive, argumentative

____ Angry, fearful

____ **Total**

Musculoskeletal

____ Muscle weakness

____ Growing pains

____ Swollen, tender joints

____ Chronic muscle or joint pain

____ **Total**

Weight

____ Water retention

____ Excessive weight

____ Binge eating

____ **Total**

Other Symptoms

____ Frequent illness

____ Premenstrual syndrome

____ Chronic urinary tract infections

____ Other _____

_____

____ **Total**

_____ **Grand Total**

© 1995 Immuno Laboratories, Inc. Reprinted with permission.

2. Adaptive Phase. *After repeated exposure to the offending food, the body will "adapt" to the negative stress and the symptoms may become less severe, shift to another part of the body, or even disappear altogether. However, the problem will not go away completely until the offending food is eliminated for a period of time. The symptoms may not reappear until years later—commonly during or after a stressful event. At this point the symptoms may be more complicated and even chronic.*

During this phase, the baby's weakened immune system will try to cope with the foreign invader (the offending food). As a result of this adaptation, the colic, diarrhea, or diaper rash will probably disappear. However, more complicated problems are on the way. As the infant grows into childhood and then becomes a teenager, the longer he or she eats the offending food, the more difficult it will become for the digestive and immune systems to manage the problem. As the strength of the immune system and liver dwindles, a number of chronic conditions, such as eczema, repeated ear or bronchial infections, hyperactivity, constipation, migraine headaches, and colitis, can develop. At this point, the family doctor is more than likely trying to treat the symptoms with medications, not realizing that the underlying cause of these symptoms is a hidden food allergy.

3. Exhaustive Phase. *After long-term exposure to the food allergy, the immune system enters the "exhaustive" phase, and becomes unable to cope with the offending food. Consequently, cells and tissues begin to deteriorate.*

As an adult, the genetically weak organs and/or systems become the primary target of deterioration and degeneration. The end result is poor digestion and the assimilation of nutrients with a totally disrupted nutrition profile. The longstanding hidden food allergies have finally worn down the immune system and resistance to disease is compromised—even death can result.

Let's take a closer look at what happens during this phase. The *antigen* (foreign substance that enters the body), stimulates the release of antibodies, which are produced by the immune system. An antibody latches onto the antigen, forming an antigen-antibody complex. As this toxin circulates through the blood, it can be deposited anywhere in the body. In the case of rheumatoid arthritis, for example, the toxins are deposited in the joints, triggering inflammation and deterioration of the joint over time. The antigen-antibody complex can trigger several other chronic illnesses, including psoriasis, multiple sclerosis, lupus, and inflammatory bowel disorders, such as Crohn's disease and ulcerative colitis.

Undiagnosed (or untreated) hidden food allergies can lead to chronic disease. Doctors of alternative medicine have known of this link for decades, and they have helped countless numbers of people become symptom free by getting to the cause of their illness—hidden food allergies. After testing nearly 3,000 patients and eliminating toxic foods from their diets, I have personally observed many remarkable recoveries from chronic health problems that had been unsuccessfully treated with drugs and surgeries for years. Food allergy testing and treatment are simple, drug-free, nonsurgical, and safe approaches for optimizing health.

If you are suffering from hidden food allergies, there is no medication, no medical treatment, and no one diet that is going to restore your health or help you lose weight (and keep it off) if you continue to eat foods that are toxic to your system.

Phony Fat

You may not be as overweight as you think. The extra fat you may be carrying around the waistline or under your chin, may be phony fat. Phony fat is not your fault. It is a consequence of hidden food allergies that you or your doctor have probably never even suspected. And the good news is that you can shed ten to twenty pounds of this deceiving weight within the first month of eliminating the allergic foods from your diet.

Phony fat can bloat your tummy, give you heartburn, cause a stuffy nose or itchy eyes, and make your face, hands, and ankles swell. If you have one or more of these symptoms, you may have phony fat. But don't fret. Once you identify and eliminate the foods that don't agree with you, you'll peel off five to ten pounds of phony fat within a couple of weeks, and possibly up to twenty pounds within the first month.

The human body is 65 to 75 percent water by weight. Even small changes in the amount of water retained can make a big difference on the bathroom scale. Hidden food allergies cause water retention, because the body perceives a reactive food as a foreign invader. Whenever a foreign invader or toxin gets inside the body, the immune system automatically tries to flush it out with water. Hormones are also released as a result of the allergic response. These hormones cause body cells and, subsequently, tissues to swell with water. Water retention looks like fat, but it is actually phony fat.

After you shed the phony fat, your body will start burning the real fat. The best news is that you will be able to keep it off permanently. Hidden food allergies slow down the body's metabolism. This promotes a sluggish thyroid gland, which disrupts hormone balance and triggers food cravings—all of which cause the body to store fat. Once you avoid the allergic foods, your metabolism will increase, thyroid

Ulcerative Colitis Cured
with an Unexpected Bonus

Sherry had a bright future as an executive secretary with a large firm until she came down with a serious case of ulcerative colitis. For over a year, Sherry's family doctor treated the condition with medication, but she got progressively worse. She had to cope with ten to fifteen bloody bowel movements each day, and she was mentally and physically exhausted. She was referred to a gastroenterologist, who prescribed several more courses of medication that failed, before recommending surgery to remove most of her large intestine. Before committing to this radical procedure, Sherry decided to call my office for a second opinion.

When I first met Sherry, she was at her wits end. Although her other doctors had told her that food had nothing to do with her condition, I suspected hidden food allergies were the cause. After an ELISA blood test revealed the offending foods, Sherry began following an allergy-free diet. Two weeks later, she was nearly symptom free. After a little more than a month, she no longer needed her medications. The intestinal bleeding and abdominal pain were almost entirely gone. She was on the road to recovery.

Six months later, Sherry was symptom-free. Her health was restored, and as a side effect, she lost over ninety pounds. She shed the unwanted pounds while eating unrestricted quantities of three of the worst carbs on the low-carb diet doctors' restricted list—potatoes, rice, and carrots—all high-glycemic carbs. Sherry now says she feels better than she has in her entire life.

Over the years, I have treated many patients with inflammatory bowel disorders like ulcerative colitis, Crohn's disease, and diverticulitis. Many of these people, just like Sherry, were told they would have to have a portion or all of their intestines removed. Instead, by simply eating an allergy-free diet consisting of carbohydrates from heaven, their intestines remained intact. And, like Sherry, many of these people lost weight without even trying.

As you can see, it is not necessary to restrict carbs to lose weight and improve health. Eating unrefined carbs that are tailor-made for each individual, allows good health and weight loss to occur naturally without counting calories or fat grams.

function will improve, and food cravings will cease. I have had hundreds of patients verify this.

You may already be eating a healthy diet. However, you may also be eating certain foods that are toxic to your body. No two people are alike—and one person's food can be another person's poison. A healthy food that may be good for your spouse could be harmful to you. Despite what some people want you to believe, no one diet fits all people. In order to feel good, lose weight, and keep it off, you need to develop an eating strategy that is tailor-made for your body.

Take Home a Tailor-Made Diet

No two people are alike—everyone has unique biochemical needs. The food you eat should be customized for your particular body chemistry. The easiest, most accurate way to identify the foods that agree, as well as disagree, with you, is through the ELISA allergy blood test. An invaluable tool in my practice, this test takes the guesswork out of identifying hidden food allergies, allowing tailor-made diets for individuals. Several diagnostic laboratories provide the ELISA allergy blood test; however, not all labs are created equal and results can vary significantly. Be sure to discuss this important consideration with your health care provider.

In addition to the ELISA blood test for determining food allergies, there are two other commonly used methods—the elimination-provocation method, and the mono-diet challenge. The *elimination-provocation method* involves writing down a list of the foods you eat more than three times a week, and then eliminating those foods for seven days. Notice if any symptoms improve during this time, or if you experience any weight loss. During the second week, begin reintroducing the foods on the list one at a time. Wait three days before reintroducing another food. Keep a diet diary (a blank form is provided on page 268) and be sure to log any symptoms that return after the introduction of a new food.

For the *mono-diet challenge,* only white rice and/or skinless potatoes (baked or boiled) are permitted for seven days. These two refined foods are nonallergenic, so eating them for a week clears the system of any by-products caused by allergic responses and their related symptoms. Foods are then reintroduced one at a time, while watching for the return of any symptoms for three days. A diet diary is kept for logging any reactions to the newly introduced foods.

As you can see, the elimination-provocation method and the mono-diet challenge are more tedious, time-consuming, and less accurate that the ELISA blood test. It is for these reasons, I recommend the ELISA blood test.

Victory Over Crippling Arthritis

George, an ambitious accountant with a young family suffered for years with a debilitating condition known as *ankylosing spondylitis*—a crippling form of arthritis. The anti-inflammatory medications that George's doctor had prescribed had become less and less effective. George's pain got progressively worse and he feared he would end up in a wheelchair. One of his biggest fears was that he would be unable to play baseball and enjoy other physical activities with his children.

Fortunately, George happened to be listening to my radio program, "The Other Side of Medicine," when he heard about the remarkable recovery of one my guests who had the same condition. He suddenly felt a sense of hope for his own condition and made appointment to see me.

George underwent a physical exam and had some blood tests done, including the ELISA food allergy test. The results showed that he was allergic to several foods, including some carbs that are common to the typical American diet. These foods were immediately removed from his diet. George began following a modified Mediterranean diet (see Chapter 8), and started taking several nutritional supplements.

Within less than three months, George no longer needed his medication and was able to walk briskly without pain. Within six months, he was symptom free. Interestingly, although George's brother, a medical doctor, also suffered from the same condition, he refused to try his brother's unconventional approach.

George's victory over illness is a classic example of how lifestyle can overpower genetic weaknesses. He took charge of his health, refusing to accept being crippled for life.

The Great Weight Debate
Too Many Carbs or Too Much Fat?

Nothing has polarized the diet world more than the current great weight debate—are Americans eating too many carbs or too much fat? Low-carb diet experts believe people are fat because they eat too many carbs. Low-fat diet experts believe people are fat because they eat too much fat. Who do you think is right?

Low-carb diet doctors claim our nation has reduced its fat intake over the past twenty-five years. They also believe it has increased its consumption of carbohydrates. Dr. Barry Sears, creator of the the Zone Diet writes, "All data analysis during the last fifteen years, shows that despite the fact that the American public has dramatically cut back on the amount of fat consumed, the country has experienced an epidemic rise in obesity." Did Sears say "data"?

According to statistics from the United States Department of Agriculture (USDA), our nation's daily fat intake has been steadily climbing. In 1970, the average American ate 107 grams of fat; in the 1980s, that number increased to 110 grams; and in 1999, it jumped to 116 grams. As you can see, the "data" clearly shows that fat consumption has been on a continuous climb.

But hold on, that's only half the problem. According to a study released in January 2004, from the Centers for Disease Control (CDC), over the last thirty years, carb consumption in America has jumped significantly. However, the study quickly points out that it is not fruits, vegetables, or whole grains that our nation is munching on. Our extra carbs—and extra pounds—are coming from sugary cookies, cakes, pies, breads, pastas, snack chips, and soft drinks that are made with refined carbs from hell.

Americans Are Eating More of Everything

The CDC reported that Americans are getting fatter because they are eating more of everything—carbs, fats, and protein. Although the government agency says carb intake is the biggest problem, they also warn that we continue to eat too much fat. It's true that the percent of calories from fat is going down, but only when compared to the percent of calories from carbs. When you crunch the numbers, we are eating more of both fat and carbs.

As it turns out, the low-carb camp and the low-fat camp are both right. As a nation, we are overweight because we are eating too many carbs and too much fat. Yet, isn't it ironic that although we are overfed, Americans are starving? The problem is that we are eating too much of the wrong type of carbs, as well as too much of the wrong types of fat. We're eating more dead calories with less nutritional value.

We are an overweight, undernourished nation that is stuffing itself with empty calories—foods deficient in vital nutrients that are needed to satisfy hunger, curb food cravings, and supply the sustained energy needed to get up and exercise. They are foods that keep you trapped in an overweight, unfit body.

Our nation needs to change its eating habits and include more dietary good guys—fruits, vegetables, beans, and whole grains. In addition, we need to take

A Nation Obsessed

The weight-loss industry is huge failure. Millions of people in ever-growing numbers become loyal subjects to a growing body of fad-diet kings. Each year, Americans spend over $40 billion on weight-loss products, plans, and diet aids. Yet surprisingly, 95 percent of those who lose weight on diets gain it back, and more.

Our nation is obsessed with dieting and weight loss. People are constantly beating themselves up with weight-loss products and fad diets. "Quick-fix" weight-loss solutions that are bound to fail, lure people into a lifetime of despair. Pills that promise you can shed pounds while you sleep, stomach stapling, diuretics, stimulants and other drugs, and fad diets are just a few of the gimmicks that Americans buy into on a daily basis in their fight against the battle of the bulge. But these people ignore the most important consideration—permanent weight loss is the outcome of a healthy lifestyle and a long-term commitment to good health. Unfortunately, the word "commitment" seems to have lost its value, yet we instinctively know that anything in life that is worthwhile takes time, effort, and commitment. Are you willing to make a commitment to a lifetime of wellness?

The road to permanent weight loss runs parallel to the road to good health. If your primary goal is to become healthy and rid yourself of headaches, fatigue, digestive problems, muscle and joint pains, and recurring illness, then weight loss will occur without even trying. Instead of making your primary goal to fit into smaller clothes, why not strive to boost your energy, strengthen your immune system, and prevent illness? Take charge of your health instead of trying to lose weight. Restoring your health will give you the power to win the battle of the bulge, and the ability to enjoy a lifetime of wellness.

advantage of essential fats from flaxseed oil, olive oil, and fish oils. These nutrient-rich oils satisfy hunger and restore and maintain health, while encouraging permanent weight loss.

The Magic of Low-Carb Diets

In *The New Diet Revolution*, Dr. Robert Atkins claims his diet has certain "metabolic advantages" that will enable you to eat as much as you want and still lose weight—as long as you restrict carbs. Is his promise true? Can dieters eat high-calorie meals and get away with losing weight because of magical "metabolic advantages?" In another best-selling low-carb book, *The Zone,* Dr. Barry Sears claims that by eating meals that are composed of 40 percent carbs, 30 percent fat, and 30 percent protein you will reach a metabolic state that will keep you thin. Readers are lead to believe that if they "enter the Zone," Sears magical metabolic state of mind and body, they will shed unwanted pounds. Has Sears discovered a set of magical numbers that can help break the weight-loss bank?

Yes, you can lose weight fast on a low-carb diet—but not because of a magical formula brewed by a best-selling author. The weight comes off for all the wrong reasons. Surprise! From Atkins "Diet Revolution" to the South Beach Diet, a reality check demonstrates that when you tally the numbers, a low-carb diet is nothing more than a low-calorie diet in disguise. That is what Stanford Medical School researcher Dr. Dena Bravata and her colleagues from Yale University discovered after conducting a review of 107 low-carb diet studies from 1966 until February 2003. The study, reported in the April 2003 issue of *The Journal of the American Medical Association,* concluded, "While these diets (low-carb) are effective in the short term, weight loss results from reduced calories, not carbohydrate restriction."

There is nothing magical about low-carb weight-loss formulas. Just think, millions of people are giving up their favorite carbs for what amounts to a calorie-restricted diet. Are you one of them? The take-home message here is that there are several safer low-calorie diets that don't restrict carbs. But the best news is that you can lose weight and keep it off on a custom diet that is individualized for you—without counting calories or restricting all carbs. If you follow the meal plan presented in Part 4, you'll be able to enjoy carbs, proteins, and fats that are compatible with your unique biochemical makeup.

Low-Carb Diets
What Are You Really Losing?

You probably didn't know it, but the rapid weight loss commonly experienced during the first month on a low-carb diet is water weight—not fat. The reason is two fold. First, carbs are made of carbon and water. Consequently, restricting carbs reduces the water retained inside the body. Second, as you have already discovered, eliminating carbs, especially grains, helps you shed pounds because they may be a source of hidden food allergies, a major cause of weight gain. Following the initial weight loss, you will lose fat on a low-carb diet, but at the rate of about a pound per week. Interestingly, this happens to be the same weight-loss rate as any calorie-restricted diet, including low-fat diets. Obviously, you don't need to restrict carbs to lose weight.

The truth is, you can lose more than just weight on a low-carb diet. First, you automatically lose the many pleasures of eating carbs. Second, and most important, you could end up losing your health. Does it make sense to lose a few extra pounds of water but sacrifice good health in the process?

Think about it. How could any one diet fit everyone? If you have tried multiple diets, medications, nutritional supplements, and exercise plans, but still can't keep the weight off, you need a diet that is designed to fit your personal nutritional needs. Once you identify and eliminate the carbs and other foods that are toxic to your body, it is possible to shed twelve to twenty pounds of extra water weight in the first month. After the first month, you'll start to lose fat while improving your health—without restricting carbs. The ELISA blood test can tell you exactly which carbs are custom-made for your body.

Is the Atkins' Diet Trimming Back the Fat?

For years, most people understood that the Atkins' Diet was an all-you-can-eat meat, cheese, and egg smorgasbord. But suddenly in 2004, the Atkins' camp started singing a different tune. According to a January 2004 story in *The New York Times,* the Atkins' Diet now recommends that only 20 percent of total daily calories come from saturated fat. Did the Atkins' organization shift its position because of outside pressure from its critics? Not according to Stuart Trager, M.D., chairman of the Atkins' Physician Council, who said, "Nothing has changed. Our message is still the same. Atkins is and always has been about controlling carbohydrates. . . . Atkins never did and still does not prescribe amounts of fats or protein. . . . Without portion restriction, this has been shown to result in weight loss." Yet, when you analyze the calorie tally on page 93, a different picture emerges. The truth is, when you eat a lot of fat, you quickly get tired of it. Consequently, you end up eating less food and, therefore, less calories.

Trager says that the 20-percent number used by Atkins' educators stems from the meal plan outlined in the Atkins' book. The diet, particularly in the induction phase, provides 60 percent of calories from fat. If you divide the diet into 20-percent polyunsaturated fat and 20-percent monounsaturated fat, the magic number of 20-percent saturated fat pops up. However, even that number is twice as much as the American Heart Association (AHA) recommends.

Surprising Calorie Tally

Although the daily intake of fat, protein, and carbohydrates on low-carb diets varies markedly from the amounts consumed on the standard American diet, the average calorie intake is lower. Calorie reduction, not carbohydrate restriction, is, in fact, one of the major reasons for weight loss on low-carb diets. This means that, at best, low-carb diets are nothing more than low-calorie diets in disguise. At worst, they pose several serious risks to good health.

DIET	AVERAGE DAILY CALORIES
Standard American	2,200
South Beach	1,500
Atkins	1,500 – 1,600
Zone	1,300 – 1,400

Robert Eckel M.D., Chairman of the AHA Nutrition, Physical Activity, and Metabolism Council, says, "I sense the cutback on saturated fat in part a political positioning in response to the South Beach Diet book, which is outselling the Atkins, *New Diet Revolution*." Isn't it interesting how quickly Atkins' marketing experts are willing to change their belief system when profit margins begin to dwindle? I wonder how Dr. Atkins would have responded.

Stop Counting Calories
Quit Dieting Forever

Although most weight-loss plans rely on portion control and calorie counting, one of the cardinal rules in my clinic (with rare exception) is that my patients don't waste their time counting calories or fat grams. Instead, I encourage them to follow these rules:

❒ Eat only when hungry.

❒ Eat to satisfaction, not to fullness.

❒ Follow a custom-made meal plan based on the findings of an ELISA allergy blood test.

❐ Follow the guidelines and principles found in the versatile and delicious American-MediterrAsian diet (presented in Part 4).

Although I'm not a weight-loss doctor, for nearly two decades, I have watched thousands of my patients lose weight without even trying. Most of these people sought my services because they suffered from a chronic illness that was not resolved by conventional medicine. For many of these people, one of the side effects of following my recommended diet and lifestyle prescription was unexpected weight loss. I want to help you receive the same benefit.

You see, my primary goal is not to help you lose weight, but rather to improve your health. I want to teach you how to take an active role in your health care so you can live a lifetime of wellness in a fit and trim body. I'll show you how to eat a delicious and satisfying plant-based diet with little emphasis on animal-based foods. I will also explain how to detoxify your liver and digestive system to improve your health and lose weight at the same time. You will discover that by simply eating the right foods, drinking lots of pure water, exercising, laughing, and playing more, you can shed those unwanted extra pounds, while saying goodbye to fatigue, aches, pains, digestive disturbances, headaches, mood swings, and much more.

We need to use more common sense. Think about all of the people around the world who are fit and trim, yet never heard of a fat gram or carb counter. How do think they maintain a healthy weight? As you will find out, the healthiest populations in the world eat carbs from heaven and live active lifestyles.

You Can Eat More and Lose Weight

I know it sounds too good to be true, but you really can eat more—without counting calories or fat grams—and still lose weight. My patients always look surprised when I tell them this, and think I've gone off the deep end. I understand their skepticism because this idea directly contradicts everything we have always been taught about weight loss. Yet, after a couple weeks on the American-MediterrAsian diet, my patients almost always return to the office with smiling faces, as they step on the scale and find themselves five, ten, or fifteen pounds lighter.

How is it possible to eat more and still lose weight? There is a logical, scientific reason for this. First of all, people have been doing it for thousands of years, so it's time-proven. Our ancestors actually ate more food than today's average American adult and weighed less. That's right. They ate more food, however, we consume more calories than they did. Researchers have discovered that because our ancestors ate only unrefined carbohydrates from heaven, they were able to eat more food while staying fit and trim. The foods our ancestors ate also had more fiber and less calories, which helped them maintain an ideal weight.

The table below shows the difference in the calorie and fiber content of a meal of carbohydrates from heaven (Heavenly Meal) and a similar meal of carbohydrates from hell (Helluva Meal). While the Heavenly Meal totaled 578 calories with 20 grams of fiber, the Helluva Meal had a whopping 1,393 calories and only 6 grams of fiber.

Helluva Meal or Heavenly Meal?

The following table shows the difference in calorie count and fiber content of two similar, yet nutritionally different meals.

HEAVENLY MEAL	PORTION	CALORIES	FIBER (GRAMS)
7-grain bun	1 bun	150	5
Southwest veggie burger	6 ounces	240	9
Tomato	1/2 cup	19	1
Lettuce	1 1/2 cups	8	1
Onions	2 slices	16	1
Baked corn chips	4 ounces	125	2
Salsa	3 ounces	20	1
Sparkling water with lemon	8 ounces	0	0
Totals		**578**	**20**
HELLUVA MEAL	**PORTION**	**CALORIES**	**FIBER (GRAMS)**
White bread bun	1 bun	175	1
Beef patty	6 ounces	550	0
Tomato	1/2 cup	19	1
Lettuce	1 1/2 cups	8	1
Onions	2 slices	16	1
French fries	4 ounces	450	2
Soda pop	12 ounces	175	0
Totals		**1,393**	**6**

The problem is that over the last 100 years, our nation has moved away from the traditional foods of our ancestors, and has come to rely on carbs from hell. Because these foods do not satisfy hunger, shortly after a meal, we are looking to eat more carbohydrates—caught in an unhealthy web.

Refined carbohydrates may taste good, but they are psychologically and physiologically addicting. Because these carbohydrates and the foods made from them weren't even around before the 1900s, our ancestors were not tempted by them. They ate only carbs from heaven, which were rich in fiber and vitamins—two of the most important factors in weight management. Although our distant relatives didn't know the foods they ate were high in fiber, low in calories, and rich in vitamins and phytochemicals, they reaped the benefits of these gifts of nature.

Can we eat refined carbs every day and simply replace the lost nutrients with fiber and other nutritional supplements? Remember, it's not nice to fool Mother Nature. Scientists have found that even if a mere 18 percent of total calories consumed come from refined carbohydrates, many of the health benefits of the fiber will be lost. There is no substitute for a diet rich in carbohydrates from heaven to help you optimize your health and lose weight.

Fiber Blocks Calorie Absorption

Scientists at the USDA found that fiber has the ability to cancel out the calories that are absorbed every day. Each gram of high-fiber carbohydrate results in a 7-calorie loss. The fiber found in fruits, vegetables, whole grains, beans, and legumes can actually block the uptake of as many as 180 calories per day. This means that by simply replacing carbs from hell with carbs from heaven, you could lose up to eighteen pounds of extra weight in a year.

Glycemic Index . . . What's Your Number, Sugar?

In the 1973 Woody Allen comedy *Sleeper,* doctors of the future refer to steak, fried foods, and fudge as healthy. They say that smoking is healthy as well. Although Allen probably never thought in his wildest imagination that this would ever be true, right now, millions of Americans are fulfilling the prophecy. A handful of low-carb diet doctors have convinced millions of Americans that they can eat all of the steak and other high saturated-fat foods they want—and it's good for them. And, of course, we all know of people who justify smoking cigarettes to curb their appetites. They fear that as soon as they quit—they will gain weight. So there you go, steak, high-fat foods, and tobacco really are today's "supposed" health foods. Woody Allen probably doesn't know it, but he's a comedian *and* a prophet.

Despite the overwhelming amount of research that demonstrates the link between heart disease and certain types of cancer with excessive amounts of saturated fat, low-carb diet doctors continue to promote high-fat diets. To further complicate the issue, they have managed to enlist the support of a number of well-credentialed doctors and scientists. Unfortunately, they have abandoned genuine science for the pseudo-science of low-carb diet doctors, who blame carbs for an increasingly overweight America. However, as you will discover, they are drawing the wrong conclusions due to flawed information and half-truths.

In all fairness, not all low-carb diet doctors recommend high levels of saturated fat, but all are quick to blame carbs for our overweight nation. Most base their weight-loss formulas in part or entirely on a scientific—but misleading—nutritional evaluation tool called the *glycemic index.*

The glycemic index (GI) is a numerical scale that is used to indicate how fast and how high specific carbohydrates raise blood glucose (sugar) levels. Originally developed as a research tool for diabetics, the glycemic index was not intended to be used for weight loss. Here is how it is calculated. Pure glucose triggers the greatest rise in blood sugar levels. Scientists standardized the glycemic index by giving glucose a set value of 100. All of the other foods are ranked on a scale of 0 to 100 according to their effect on blood sugar levels in comparison to glucose (some sugar responses can go even higher). Ranked between 0 and 45, *low-glycemic* foods raise blood sugar levels gradually, providing a slow, steady release of sugar for sustained energy. Foods in the *moderate-glycemic* range fall between 45 and 60, and produce a medium surge of sugar. Foods that are *high-glycemic* rank above 60, and create a quick spike in blood sugar levels that results in rebound hunger.

The popular book *Sugar Busters* states, "Knowledge of the glycemic index is a key to understanding the Sugar Busters Diet," which claims it can help you "lose weight, lower cholesterol, achieve optimal wellness, increase energy, and help treat diabetes and other diseases." The book *The Glucose Revolution* claims the ". . . glycemic index can help you not only to lose weight, but also reduce your risk of heart disease, improve your athletic performance, manage diabetes, and enjoy total wellness." The Atkins' and the South Beach Diets use it as a measuring stick for identifying good and bad carbs. The glycemic index has become a household word for millions of dieters, but is it a reliable tool for weight loss?

Low-carb diets that use the glycemic index to determine the good and bad carbs sound legitimate because the index is based on scientific research. But science has limitations, and so does the glycemic index, which makes many of the foods we were warned to avoid for years look like health foods, while making other foods we were told to eat without reservation, look bad.

Does the glycemic index have value? In the hands of a research scientist, the index certainly has merit. In the hands of a physician or nutritionist who doesn't understand its limitations, the glycemic index may be used improperly and provide misleading information. A basic understanding of the glycemic index will help prevent you from being misled by diets that use it to support their formulas.

Glycemic Index—Facts and Flaws

I first learned about the glycemic index in 1988 at a nutrition seminar for health care professionals. When I looked at one of the charts, my gut-level reaction was, "I don't believe it!" How could a nutritional evaluation tool that rates a Snickers bar, a Twix chocolate-caramel cookie, and ice cream as healthier choices than whole wheat bread, brown rice, or a banana have any value? It sounded crazy. Even though the instructor and the other doctors attending the seminar were intrigued by the glycemic index, I was not. I thought it would fail as a dietary assessment tool—I was wrong. In fact, it has been widely used by health care practitioners for many years. But the truth is that many doctors are misleading their patients because of their incomplete understanding of the glycemic index. And the recommendations they provide as a result may be harmful.

Despite its many flaws, the glycemic index has played a major role in the development of the low-carb diet craze. It is a controversial tool even among researchers. In an effort to clear up some of the confusion, it's important to understand some of its flaws.

Take a look at the Glycemic Index Food Table on the next page. The ranking of *some* listed foods according to the index does make sense. For example, apples have a low glycemic index (GI) rank of 38, and white sugar has a high GI of 65. Nothing we don't already know—apples are healthy; white sugar should be handled with caution. But the GI numbers for some other foods are absolutely outlandish and can confuse even the best doctors and nutritionists, not to mention the average person who is trying to decide which foods to eat.

Glycemic Index Food Table

The following list includes a sampling of the foods found on the glycemic index—a numerical scale for indicating how fast and how high specific carbohydrates raise blood sugar levels. The lower the number, the slower and more gradually the food raises blood sugar levels, providing a slow, steady release of sugar. However, the glycemic index has a number of flaws that can cause it to be misleading (see the information beginning on the previous page).

LOW (0 TO 45)		MODERATE (46 TO 60)		HIGH (61 AND ABOVE)	
Peanuts	15	Vanilla cake with frosting	42	Shredded wheat	62
Barley, pearled	25	Grape-Nuts, Post	46	Coca-Cola	63
Black beans	30	Oatmeal	49	Beets, canned	64
Lentils	30	Kiwi	52	White sugar	65
Peach	30	Sweet potato	54	Pineapple	66
Soy milk	31	Mango	55	Cornmeal	68
Apple	38	Banana	55	Bread, whole wheat	69
Navy beans	38	Brown rice	55	White bread	70
Chocolate fudge cake with frosting	38	Frosted Flakes, Kellogg's	55	Watermelon	72
Pear	38	Pita bread, whole wheat	57	Jellybeans	80
Snickers bar	41	Bran muffin	60	Potato, baked	85
Orange, navel	44			Carrots	90
Twix bar	44			Dates, dried	103

For instance, whole wheat bread has a GI of 69, while sugar-frosted flakes cereal has GI of 55. Not only does the glycemic index make it seem that whole wheat bread, carrots, a baked potato, and numerous other natural foods are not as healthy for you as sugar-frosted flakes, it also puts a Snickers bar at a GI of 41 and a Twix bar at a GI of 44, ahead of them! Even a child knows this can't be right! With numbers like these, it wouldn't be hard to convince overweight kids to use this diet tool. Which kid wouldn't like to choose jellybeans, with a GI of 80, over carrots, with a GI of 90?

Here's another problem. The glycemic index does not take into account the positive effects of fiber. In other words the index does not take the whole food into consideration. This may misrepresent how much a food will actually affect blood sugar levels in real life. Let me explain. The glycemic index score is a measurement of an individual's blood sugar response after eating 50 grams of carbohydrates in a laboratory setting. But in real life, the amount of digestible carbohydrates an individual actually eats may be much less, or much more. For instance, there is a lot more bulk in 50 grams of carbohydrate from carrots or squash than there is in a soft drink or a candy bar.

Vegetables contain a large portion of indigestible fiber, which provides a feeling of fullness, but does not affect blood sugar or contain calories. This means, for example, in order to get 50 grams of carbohydrates from carrots, you would need to eat one-and-a-quarter pounds—approximately seven carrots. Nobody eats that many carrots, except Bugs Bunny. In real life, you may eat only one carrot at a meal, which is approximately 7 grams of carbohydrate. What about winter squash? To get 50 grams of carbohydrate from winter squash, you would have to eat one-and-three-quarter pounds. My goodness! You could feed a whole family with that amount.

On the other hand, sweet treats made with carbs from hell contain almost all digestible carbohydrates, lots of calories, and no fiber. With these foods (if you want to call them "foods"), 50 grams of carbohydrates add up real fast. For example, one Snickers bar or one can of sugar-sweetened soda contains about twelve teaspoons of table sugar, which provides 50 grams of carbohydrates. And it's certainly not uncommon for people to eat one or two candy bars or drink a couple of sodas at one sitting. The chart on page 101 presents more examples.

Another major problem with the glycemic index is that it doesn't take calories into account, and the number of calories found in various foods with the same glycemic rating can differ significantly. For example, potatoes, carrots, white bread, and white sugar all have a high glycemic index. However, per pound, carrots have a skimpy 190 calories and white potatoes have 440, while the white bread calorie count is a whopping 1,300, and white sugar is an outrageous 1,700! Obviously, these foods are not equal culprits in the battle of the bulge. White sugar has an unbelievable 895 percent higher calorie count than carrots.

Another glycemic index deficiency is that it does not measure insulin levels. Yet, popular low-carb diets assume that if a food has a high-glycemic rating, it automatically means that food has an equally high insulin response. Low-carb diet experts also assume that since high-protein foods have a low-glycemic index, they automatically have the same effect on insulin. But the truth is, proteins raise insulin levels, and some proteins raise them significantly; yet low-carb diet doctors blindly favor high-protein foods over carbohydrates like fruits, vegetables, and whole grains.

I think you get the picture. The glycemic index ignores the whole food, including the bulk or mass of the food and the energy density (calories per pound). Researchers also warn that the glycemic index values are not absolute. Each food's effect on blood sugar levels depends upon several factors, including the ripeness of the food, the quantity, how long it was cooked, and the glycemic index of other foods in the meal. It must also take into account the person's recent activity level, as well as his or her insulin level.

It all boils down to this. In a strict laboratory setting, potatoes, carrots, brown rice, and other good carbs have high-glycemic numbers; in real life, these foods encourage weight loss. Why? Because they are high in fiber and have a mild impact on blood sugar and insulin levels. The low-carb camp claims just the opposite, and those who are trying to drop a few extra pounds don't realize they're being misled.

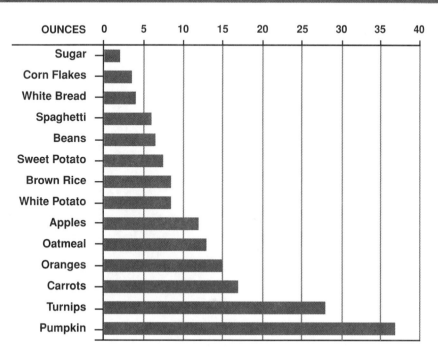

Source: USDA nutrient database for standard reference, Release 12

The Devil's Sweet Deal

Food processors cut a sweet deal with the devil when they added another evil ingredient to carbs from hell—high fructose corn syrup. Start reading food labels and you'll quickly discover this inexpensive sweetener is everywhere, from soft drinks and boxed cereals to ketchup and canned soups. Back in 1970, Americans ate about eight ounces of high fructose corn syrup per person every year. According to a study published in the *American Journal of Clinical Nutrition*, by the end of 1990, that number jumped to an unbelievable sixty-two pounds—an extra 228 calories per day. Not surprisingly, during that same twenty-year time span, the country's obesity rate more than doubled.

Fructose decreases the production of *leptin*, a hormone that shuts off switches in the brain that control appetite. Consequently, if your diet contains too much fructose, you'll end up overeating and gaining weight. (See page 104 for a more detailed discussion of leptin.) According to Peter Havel, Ph.D., a nutrition researcher at the University of California, Davis, "Fructose is more readily metabolized into fat." Havel and other researchers believe there is a strong connection between fructose in the American diet and the country's obesity epidemic. Obviously, what is helping fatten the bank accounts of the soft-drink and fast-food industries is also helping fatten Americans. Fructose also promotes insulin resistance, a growing problem that increases the risk for heart disease.

Don't be concerned with the small amounts of fructose found in honey or fresh fruit. These foods are balanced with a powerhouse of nutrients. Rather, beware of the cheap fructose sweeteners within our food supply that have enabled food giants to supersize their portions. Greg Critser, a journalist and author of *Fat Land*, explains, "The serving size of sodas has almost doubled, from about 10 ounces to about 18 ounces." Supersizing foods with fructose has provided the food manufacturers a bundle of money to deposit in their bank accounts while you deposit more fat around your waistline. Meddling with our food supply may be a sweet deal for the devil and the food manufacturers, but any time you fall for it, you're going to get burned.

Glycemic Paradox

Low-carb diet doctors may convince people to follow their eating strategy by using pseudo science, but they can't spin the success of traditional diets, which have withstood the test of time. For example although the traditional Asian diet is 65 to 75 percent carbohydrates, those who follow it have the lowest incidence of obesity and heart disease in the world. Interestingly, their main dietary staple is rice—a high-glycemic food that low-carb advocates believe triggers weight gain.

Some people may argue that the Asian population is genetically equipped to burn carbohydrates more efficiently. Research, however, proves otherwise. Several population studies have tracked healthy Asian people who ate their traditional diets and had a low incidence of obesity, diabetes, heart disease, and cancer. As these individuals migrated to the United States and abandoned their traditional diet for standard American fare, their rate of obesity, heart disease, and cancer increased dramatically—to the same level of those who were born in the United States.

Another similar pattern is found with the Pima Indians, whose diet and health patterns have been studied by scientist for the past several decades. The Pima Indians are indigenous to Mexico, but part of the tribe migrated to Arizona. Although both tribes are genetically the same, their diets and health are significantly different. The Pima of Arizona, who abandoned their traditional lifestyle and diet for the standard American diet and way of life, are plagued with a high incidence of illness—the direct result of a diet that includes excessive amounts of refined carbohydrates and saturated fat. On the other hand, the Pima of Mexico, who still follow the traditional diet and lifestyle that their ancestors relied on for centuries, continue to enjoy good health.

Scientists have labeled the vast differences between the health patterns of the two tribes the *Pima paradox*. Over half the adult population of the Pima of Arizona who are over age fifty, have type II diabetes. They also have a high incidence of heart disease. Yet, the Pima of Mexico have a less than 2-percent incidence of diabetes, obesity, and heart disease, which occurs primarily in the elderly. Scientists have also observed that the Pima of Arizona engage in less than two hours of physical activity per week, compared to the twenty-three hours exhibited by the Mexican tribe. Obviously, the diet and lifestyle of these two populations is different. Hopefully, the Pima of Arizona will soon return to their traditional diet and lifestyle, and regain their health.

Since these two populations emerged from the same genetic pool, researchers have been able to gain a rich understanding of the interplay between genetics and lifestyle. The Pimas are historically fit and trim, as long as they adhere to their traditional diets and lifestyle. Adopting the American diet and lifestyle awakened their genetic weaknesses. Consequently, obesity is out of control in the Pimas of Arizona.

The take-home message of the Pima paradox and the glycemic index is that carbohydrates are not the cause of obesity, diabetes and heart disease. The diet of the Pima of Mexico includes potatoes, carrots, and corn—all high-glycemic foods. Yet, obesity, diabetes, heart disease, and cancer are almost nonexistent within their culture. Millions of people have drawn the wrong conclusion about carbs because of the misleading information provided by low-carb diet doctors. The truth is, carbs don't make you fat—the standard American diet and lifestyle do.

Boost Leptin and Curb Your Appetite

As previously mentioned, leptin, a hormone that is stored and released from the fat cells in both animals and humans, helps to curb appetite and rev up the body's metabolism to burn fat. The Pima of Mexico take advantage of this critical appetite-control hormone, and now you can too! You see, leptin is remarkably easy to stimulate (although most doctors don't know how). Back in 1995, there was a nationwide flurry of interest in this hormone when scientists discovered that injecting it into mice triggered significant weight loss. To the dismay of every dieter and drug company, leptin treatments in humans failed miserably and this hormone quickly lost its favor.

Although drug companies can't create a pill to take advantage of leptin's appetite-curbing benefits, you can—with the food you put on your plate. Researchers believe that a low-fat, high-fiber diet, like that of the traditional Pima Indian, not only boosts leptin levels, but also makes it more active and efficient. On the other hand, high-fat diets suppress and deactivate leptin, rendering it less efficient. You can make the leptin in your bloodstream work more efficiently to boost weight loss. Take a lesson from the Pima Indians.

Satiety Index and Insulin Score

The Satiety Index (SI) and Insulin Score are two diet-assessment tools that are almost always overlooked by low-carb diet doctors. Trying to use the glycemic index to evaluate a food's effect on weight while ignoring these two diet tools is a big mistake.

The Satiety Index measures how full or satisfied a person feels during the two-hour period after eating a set amount of calories (240) from specific foods. White bread is used as the baseline of 100. Any food that scores over 100 is more satisfying than white bread; foods ranked lower are less satisfying. High-ranked foods are those with fewer calories and more filling. Guess which food ranks the highest. Surprise! It is the potato—the high-glycemic food considered to be a villain by low-carb diet doctors.

Foods with high fiber and water content, like whole grains, beans, legumes, fruits, and vegetables, rate high on the Satiety Index. High-fat, low-fiber foods rank low. Susanna Holt, Ph.D., the scientist who developed the Satiety Index says, "We think the reason is that fat is seen by the body as a fuel which should be used only in emergencies—it stores it in the cells, instead of breaking it down for immediate use. Because it doesn't recognize the fat as energy for immediate use, the body does not tell the brain to cut hunger signals, so we go on wanting more. Carbohydrates are the opposite—they raise blood glucose so the body knows it has gotten enough fuel."

A doughnut scored a low 68, while a baked/boiled potato with the skin scored 323—three times more filling than white bread—although French fries scored a low 117. Whole wheat bread was found to be twice as filling as white bread. Foods like cookies, cakes, and doughnuts made with carbohydrates from hell, turned out to be the least filling and containing the most calories. So the truth is, if you are trying to lose weight, potatoes are one of one of the best choices for satisfying those hunger pangs. Doughnuts, on the other hand, are right out of hell and will have you looking for more food in no time at all.

So as you can see, foods that are high in fiber and low in fat are more filling, have fewer calories, and satisfy hunger for longer periods of time. My great-tasting American-MediterrAsian diet provides all of these benefits—and you don't have to count calories or keep track of glycemic index scores while following it.

When all is said and done, losing weight boils down to a simple mathematical formula: "calories in" versus "calories out." If the number of calories you eat (calories in) is less than the amount of calories you burn during physical activity (calories out), you will lose weight. But this doesn't mean you have to count calories at mealtime—as long as you eat carbohydrates from heaven. Remember, carbs from heaven have a low-calorie, high-fiber content. And because fiber is not digestible, it doesn't add one calorie to your tally. This means you can eat more food with fewer calories and lose weight in the process. Fruits, vegetables, beans, and whole grains, allow you to leave the table feeling satisfied without breaking the calorie bank.

Despite claims made by the low-carb diet camp, carbohydrates have more of an impact on satiety (fullness) than fat. Fiber is one of the key elements that can boost this feeling of fullness. Some fibers are better at it than others. Water-insoluble fiber in foods like whole wheat bread, whole wheat pasta, and vegetables increases fullness for the short term (a couple hours). Water-soluble fiber found in apples, pears, unrefined oats, barley, beans, and lentils has more staying power, and can produce a feeling of fullness many hours after a meal.

Insulin Score—how high a food raises your insulin level—is an other dietary assessment tool. One of the main arguments that low-carb diet doctors use to support their diet is that carbs raise blood sugar levels, which, in turn elevate insulin levels. Insulin is a hormone that acts like a key to unlock the door to all cells and allow both carbs (as glucose) and protein (as amino acids) to enter. And in theory, elevated insulin levels are responsible for making us fat. Is this right?

Actually, this theory represents only part of the truth. In this particular instance, low-carb diets implicate carbs as the *only* foods that raise insulin levels. But in reality, both carbs *and* protein trigger the release of insulin to transport glucose and amino acids into the cells. As a matter of fact, *some protein foods raise insulin levels higher than carbs.* Beef, lamb, pork, chicken, and turkey, for instance, raise insulin levels 27 percent higher than whole wheat pasta noodles. Most dairy products raise the level almost as high as white bread does. The bottom line is that protein as well as carbohydrates raise insulin levels.

Incidentally, a food's glycemic index score does not always correlate with the Insulin Score. Every food varies in the amount of carbs, protein, and fat it contains—and each of these three macronutrients has an influence on the insulin response and score.

The low-carb diet, according to Dr. Dean Ornish, well-known internist and highly vocal critic of this diet, is concerned that Americans are not getting the true picture of the low-carb diet, which he considers "a diet of half-truths." He also says, "You can lose weight on Phen-Phen, but that doesn't mean that it's good for you. When you go on a high-protein diet, you may temporarily lose weight—but you may also mortgage your health in the process."

Obesity and Insulin Levels

Carbs from heaven actually help reduce the burden that insulin exerts on the body, because they do not create a heavy demand for its production. On the other hand, carbs from hell stimulate the overproduction of insulin. Consuming them causes a rapid spike in blood sugar levels, which causes the body to produce insulin. Since the average American eats an inordinate amount of refined white sugar, flour, pasta, and other carbs from hell, insulin levels are constantly spiking throughout the day.

The relationship between insulin and obesity is controversial. Some researchers have observed that increased levels of insulin circulating in the blood may be a cause of obesity. This theory is logical because insulin does trigger the production and storage of body fat. Further evidence to support this theory stems from the fact that type II diabetics, who are typically obese, usually have excess insulin circulating in their blood. On the other side of the theoretical fence, a significant body of research indicates that being overweight is what triggers high insulin levels.

One thing is certain—carbs from heaven minimize the body's production of insulin. Whether they help you to lose weight because of this or because they contain fewer calories is irrelevant. The bottom line is if you eat carbs from heaven and eliminate carbs from hell, you will lose weight.

Summing It Up

I find it interesting that for thousands of years only those who were affluent could afford to include excessive quantities of meat and foods made with refined carbohydrates in their diets. Before World War II, most people didn't have the means to readily obtain these foods, yet they desired to have them, just like the rich. Now that everyone can afford them, the tables have turned. A large percentage of the affluent population has abandoned its unhealthy dietary habits, choosing instead to eat unrefined carbs and little or no meat. As more and more people are becoming increasingly health conscious and aware of the truth, they are realizing that traditional peasant diets will enable them to live fuller, healthier lives, while staying fit and trim at the same time.

Chapter Seven

Fighting Heart Disease and Cancer

Cardiovascular disease is the number-one cause of death in the United States. Currently, 69 million Americans suffer with high blood pressure, high cholesterol, clogged arteries, and other diseases of the heart and blood vessels. Each year, about 1.5 million American adults will have a heart attack—1 million will die. Another 300,000 people will die from strokes caused by plaque in the arteries.

Compared to other leading causes of death in the United States, heart disease kills an exceptionally high number of people. For example, cancer claims the lives of nearly 500,000 people each year. That's less than 60 percent of those who die from diseases of the heart and blood vessels. About 30,000 people die from AIDS—around 1.5 percent less.

Many doctors and their patients continue to blame heart disease on genetics and the aging process. Yet researchers are becoming more convinced that diet and lifestyle are the primary causes. Scientists have known for some time that several populations have a very low incidence of heart disease, as long as they eat their traditional plant-based diets. However, when these same people adopt a high-fat, refined-carbohydrate diet, their incidence of heart disease increases dramatically. The Japanese, for instance, have always had an extremely low incidence of heart disease. But, as they migrated to the United States and adopted our diet and lifestyle, their heart disease rate increased significantly.

Heart disease is a recent epidemic. It was once so rare that the first report of its existence was published in *The Journal of the American Medical Association* in 1912. During that time, Dr. Paul Dudley White, a famous surgeon, had to search for ten years to find just three cases of the disease. Today, heart disease plagues millions of people in cities both large and small across the United States.

A Plant-Based Diet Reverses Heart Disease

There is substantial evidence proving that diet and lifestyle are the causes of most cardiovascular diseases. Still, most physicians only scratch the nutritional surface to help reverse this number-one cause of death in America. Most heart disease can be prevented and even cured without drugs or surgery. Although several factors contribute to the prevention and reversal of heart disease, diet plays a major role and should be one of the most important considerations. Science is just now heeding the wisdom of several old-world cultures that prevent heart disease simply by following their traditional plant-based diets.

Dr. Dean Ornish, an internist and member of the teaching staff at University of California San Francisco School of Medicine, is a pioneer in the prevention and treatment of heart disease. A frequent speaker at medical conventions, including those of the American Heart Association, Dr. Ornish, is now proving that a plant-based diet can even reverse severe heart disease. He has developed the only diet and heart-treatment program that is scientifically proven to reverse heart disease without drugs or surgery. This program is now being used as an alternative to bypass surgery in several hospitals in the United States. It has helped thousand of patients reduce or eliminate angina pain and reverse blockages in the coronary arteries. It has also allowed them to reduce or discontinue their use of medications, while feeling more energized and yet calm.

According to *Newsweek*, "Dr. Ornish's work could change the lives of millions. At the end of the year, most patients reported that their chest pains had virtually disappeared—for 82 percent of the patients, arterial clogging had reversed. They started to feel better almost immediately, and today they feel great. Dr. Ornish's patients are thrilled with their new lives. By the standards of conventional medicine, the impossible has happened." A plant-based diet can actually reverse the damage caused by a high-fat, high-protein diet. Anyone considering a low-carb, high-protein diet should seriously think about this.

Bypassing the Bypass

According to the *American Journal of Cardiology*, almost 80 percent of the people who were eligible for bypass surgery or angioplasty were able to safely avoid it by following Dr. Ornish's plant-based, low-protein diet.

Dr. Ornish's book *Reversing Heart Disease* is a must-read for anyone with heart disease. In it, Dr. Ornish states, "We found almost a 40-percent reduction in LDL-cholesterol in people who made the dietary and lifestyle changes we recommend, angina decreased by 91 percent (usually within a few weeks), myocardial perfusion increased dramatically, and coronary artery lesions showed some regression after one year and even more regression after five years."

According to Dr. Ornish, the low-fat, high-carbohydrate traditional diet of the Asian peasant population—coupled with its low rate of heart disease—is the rationale for his treatment plan. In the United States, where one-third of the calories are derived from fat, the heart disease death rate is twenty times higher than the rate found in the population of rural China. He also points to the low incidence of obesity, diabetes, and many cancers among world population groups with very low-fat, high-carbohydrate diets.

Anyone who is considering bypass surgery, should look into Dr. Ornish's program, which is offered in several hospitals across the country. Many major medical plans now pay for this treatment option, which can help prevent unnecessary suffering, not to mention the very high cost of bypass operations. In one of Dr. Ornish's recent interviews, he said, "Stable patients are often told, 'Mr. Jones or Miss Smith, your choice is that you can have a bypass or you can die' when, in fact, for most of those people there is no evidence that a bypass or angioplasty is going to prolong their life."

As good as Dr. Ornish's program is, many doctors and nutritionists, including me, do not think it is necessary to restrict certain fats to prevent or reverse heart disease. Yes, the incidence of heart disease is low in rural China; however, it is also low in the Mediterranean population, where fat consumption can be as high as 40 percent in total calorie intake. The difference between healthy Greek peasants, and illness-prone Americans is not the quantity of the fat they consume, but rather the type.

Americans eat significantly more saturated fats, found in meat and dairy products, than both their Asian and Mediterranean counterparts. The standard American diet is also high in hydrogenated fats found in margarine, refined vegetable oils, and packaged convenience foods. These foods are not found in the traditional Mediterranean diet, which is rich in healthy fats like monounsaturated fats found in olive oil, and polyunsaturated and omega-3 fats found in fish, vegetables, and whole grains.

Syndrome X

Syndrome X can accelerate the aging process, cause your waistline to take the shape of an apple, and set the stage for multiple chronic diseases. Millions of Americans already have it—and you may be one of them. What is this mysterious sounding condition? Syndrome X is a cluster of symptoms that includes insulin resistance, (inability to absorb sugar from the blood), high blood pressure, high cholesterol, high triglycerides, and increased weight—especially around the waist. These risk factors are further detailed in the table on page 113. Syndrome X increases an individual's risk for diabetes, heart disease, and stroke. Dr. Gerald Reavan, Stanford Medical School endocrinologist, first introduced the term Syndrome X during the 1988 annual convention of the American Diabetic Association. Reaven states, "The more risk factors you have, and the more severe they are, the greater your risk of a heart attack, a stroke and diabetes. Yet despite the serious nature of this common disorder, it may go unrecognized by your doctor."

Researchers have found high insulin levels and insulin resistance as the common factors among all of the symptoms of Syndrome X. Both insulin resistance and the more serious progression of this common disorder, Syndrome X, do have a common genetic predisposition. However, most of the blame for both conditions is not attributed to genetics, but rather to excessive amounts of refined carbohydrates and saturated fats in the diet. Syndrome X is a disease of overconsumption. It's a "plague of plenty," triggered by an overabundance of carbohydrates from hell and the wrong kind of fats.

According to Christie Ballantyne, M.D., director of the Center for Cardiovascular Disease Prevention at Baylor College of Medicine and The Methodist DeBakey Heart Center in Houston, "The problem is that doctors still focus on total cholesterol as the main indicator of heart disease risk." States Ballantyne, "They don't understand that a patient can have a total cholesterol of two hundred, average for an American, yet have a dangerous case of metabolic syndrome."

Do You Have An Apple Figure?

An apple a day may keep the doctor away, but an apple shape around your waistline means there is a good chance you may soon be visiting your doctor with a heart problem. Scientists warn that distribution of body fat makes obesity even more dangerous—and it can determine your risk for heart disease. It is not just total body fat that counts. Weight that settles into the midline area, creating an "apple-shaped" body, is one of the risk factors associated with Syndrome X. This type of fat distribution is more common in men; however, it also occurs in women, especially after menopause.

Do you have an apple figure? Either determine your waist-to-hip ratio or simply measure your waistline. To determine your waist-to-hip ratio, first measure the distance around your waist just about an inch above the belly button. Next, measure the widest point around your hips. Then, divide your waist measurement by your hip measurement. A number 0.8 or higher for women, and 1.0 or higher for

Risk Factors for Syndrome X

Any cluster that includes at least three of the following symptoms is characteristic of Syndrome X.

RISK FACTOR	DEFINING LEVELS
Abdominal obesity (apple-shape)	Men: waist size > 40 inches Women: waist size > 35 inches
Triglyceride level	150 or higher
HDL-cholesterol	Men: < 40 Women: < 50
Blood pressure	Systolic: 130 or higher Diastolic: 85 or higher
Fasting glucose level	110 or higher

Source: National Institutes of Health, NHLBI, ATP III Guidelines At-a-Glance Quick Desk Reference 2001.

men indicates an apple-shaped figure. If you don't want to go through the trouble of calculating this ratio, simply measure your waistline. A waistline greater than 40 inches in men and 35 inches in women indicates a risk for developing Syndrome X.

Researchers agree that proper diet and lifestyle choices are optimum treatments for Syndrome X. But most doctors have little training in nutrition, so they end up prescribing superficial dietary modifications that fail. Consequently, millions of people with "apple figures" are left on their own to figure out what to eat. Many turn to low-carb diets.

Low-carb diet doctors are partially right—we *are* eating too many carbs and not enough fat, but they are carbohydrates from hell and not enough essential fats. In order to prevent or overcome Syndrome X, you need to replace saturated fat with essential fats, and refined carbs with unrefined carbs. The American-Mediterr-Asian diet found in Part 4, provides recipes that include both. By following this diet, you will be able to enjoy carbohydrates from heaven like potatoes, brown rice, whole wheat products, beans, and legumes, along with the benefits of essential fats found in olive oil, canola oil, nuts, avocados, and cold-water fish. You can eat more fat—good fat. And you don't have to give up your favorite carbs to lose weight. These foods will help make your cells more sensitive to insulin, prevent the onset of Syndrome X, and help you stay trim and fit as a fiddle.

Are You Still Confused About Fat?

For the past few years, an acceptable range of LDL "bad" cholesterol was set for all Americans—yet every thirty seconds, at least one person experiences a heart attack, and every minute someone dies from one. One thing became clear: people's dietary habits were not on the proper path for good health. In an effort to change the country's eating patterns (and reduce the statistics of America's number-one health problem), health officials recently lowered acceptable LDL levels based upon a person's risk category. Although the new guidelines are a step in the right direction, they can be effective only through a clear understanding of dietary fats.

Between the 1950s and 1970s, Americans knew only one thing about fat—it made food taste good! Back then, it was common to spread butter on everything—from popcorn to ham sandwiches. High-fat buttermilk and "marbled meats" were desirable. But once the word got out that high-fat diets were linked to heart disease and cancer, fat became a complicated issue.

It turns out that some fats are heart healthy, others are not. For example, an excess of saturated fat and cholesterol, which is found in animal foods, causes circulation disorders and heart disease. Although doctors once told us that margarine was heart healthy—in reality, it causes clogged arteries. The USDA Food Guide Pyramid (detailed in Chapter 8) suggests we should limit all fats. But a mound of research has proven monounsaturated fat, found in extra-virgin olive oil, cold-pressed canola oil, avocados, walnuts, almonds, pecans, and macadamia nuts, actually helps prevent heart disease. Omega-3 fats found in flaxseeds, walnuts, pumpkin seeds, dark leafy green vegetables, and cold-water fish help to reduce inflammation—a major risk factor for heart disease.

Then there is cholesterol. To borrow a term coined by comedian Jerry Seinfeld, "What's the deal with cholesterol?" Most people know one thing—too much cholesterol is not good. But before explaining why, it's important to understand some cholesterol basics. Our body needs cholesterol, which is contained in the outer wall of every cell. Cholesterol is necessary to make hormones and vitamin D, as well as aid in the digestion of fats. Our bodies depend on it. In fact, the liver makes all the cholesterol we need. But that's where the problem begins. If we eat too many foods that contain cholesterol, we end up getting too much of a good thing. Excess cholesterol floating around in the blood is converted into fat. Even worse, when cholesterol is heated or dried, it reacts with oxygen and becomes oxidized. This dangerous form of cholesterol can accumulate in the arteries as plaque. Oxidized cholesterol, in combination with inflammation that stems from infections, obesity, poor diet, and even gum disease, can weaken the plaque formed on the blood vessel walls. Under the right circumstances, the plaque can rupture, block the circulation of blood, and cause a heart attack or stroke.

Angelic Fats and Lucifer's Lipids

What about good and bad cholesterol? HDL is good and LDL is bad. Or is it the other way around? Many people struggle with these two terms. Here's an easy way to remember —the "H" in HDL (good) cholesterol, stands for "heavenly," while the "L" in LDL (bad) cholesterol, stands for "Lucifer," the fallen angel.

HDL cholesterol is good because it mops up cholesterol in the blood, sends it back to the liver, which then expels it from the body. Then there is LDL cholesterol. Even though LDLs are considered "evil" substances, we need them to deliver essential cholesterol throughout the body. The problem begins with too much LDL cholesterol—or oxidized LDL cholesterol.

Fiber Lowers Cholesterol Better than Statin Drugs

Like a clean-up crew that picks up debris after a party, fiber found in carbs from heaven acts like a clean-up crew that picks up and eliminates cholesterol from the body. Research scientists have known for years that fiber lowers cholesterol. However, it is important to know that only water-soluble fiber can mop up and flush cholesterol out of the body. Water-soluble fiber is found in fruits, vegetables, oats, barley, beans, legumes, and nuts—carbohydrates from heaven.

Eating some of these fiber-rich foods every day will help reduce total cholesterol and triglyceride levels, increase HDL cholesterol, and lower LDL cholesterol. Here is how it works. Inside the intestines, cholesterol hitches a ride on the back of water-soluble fiber, which carries it from the body in the stool. If there is not enough water-soluble fiber available, the leftover cholesterol will be reabsorbed into the blood. Dietary fiber helps decrease the production of cholesterol in the liver. It also helps reduce the concentration of the bile salts that are produced in the liver, which, in turn, helps to prevent the formation of gallstones.

Statin drugs, such as Zocor, Lipitor, and Pravachol, may lower cholesterol, but they are risky business. Fiber, on the other hand, lowers cholesterol while reducing the overall risk of heart attack without any dangerous side effects. Treat your body right. Instead of popping a pill to lower cholesterol, try eating more fiber—eat carbohydrates from heaven.

Several large studies have demonstrated that a plant-based diet of unrefined carbs, which are rich in dietary fiber, can significantly lower the risk for heart disease. In one study involving over 40,000 males, Harvard research scientists found that a high-fiber diet was associated with a 40-percent lower risk of heart disease, compared to those individuals with a low-fiber intake. The researchers noted that the water-soluble fiber found in grains, like oats, appeared to have the greatest benefit. In another study, published in a 1999 issue of *The Journal of the American Medical Association*, researchers reported that women in the Harvard Nurses' Health Study who ate at least two-and-a-half servings of whole grains per day had a 30-percent lower risk of developing heart disease than the women who ate less than one serving per week.

Flaxseeds, one of the best available sources of water-soluble fiber and essential oils, helps reduce cholesterol. Its nutty flavor complements many dishes. You can buy them whole or ground (you can grind them yourself in a coffee grinder) and sprinkle them on cereal and salads. Flax flour (made from de-fatted flaxseeds) boosts the nutritional content of baked goods. It has a large amount of water-soluble fiber and plant lignans—but no oil. Flaxseed oil is good in salads and drizzled over cooked foods.

Carbohydrates and Cancer

About 1.5 million people in America are diagnosed with cancer each year—that's one out of every three people. Over 500,000 die from it. The National Academy of Sciences estimates that 60 percent of all cancers in women, and 40 percent in men are due to dietary risk factors. According to these statistics, on average, we could prevent over 250,000 cancer-related deaths and over 750,000 cancer cases from developing every year, simply by making the right food choices.

We spend billions of dollars on high-tech diagnostic procedures and treatments for cancer, but less than 2 percent of our health-care budget is spent on education for cancer prevention. Dr. Phillip Lee, Professor of Social Medicine and Director of the Health Policy Program, University of California, San Francisco, had this to say, "As a nation, we have come to believe that medicine and medical technology can solve our major health problems. The role of such important factors as diet in cancer and heart disease has long been obscured by the emphasis on conquering these diseases through the miracles of modern medicine. Treatment, not prevention, has been the order of the day. But the problem can never be solved merely by more and more medical care."

Cancer Research "The Future Is Food"

In an article discussing the future of cancer research in the November 1998 issue of *Newsweek*, Dr. Mitchell Gaynor, head oncologist at New York's Strang-Cornell Cancer Prevention Center, said, "We have seen the future, and the future is food."

The problem is, we receive too much conflicting information on diet and cancer. It's no wonder so many people take the attitude: "Forget about it. Why should I even bother?" But throwing your hands up in frustration won't protect you from the reality that cancer can strike you or a loved one. And besides, are you really willing to give up the power you have to control your risk of developing this disease? The right foods have the power to help prevent cancer, and you are the one who controls the power. Let's take a look at some of the facts on diet and cancer.

In 1997, the American Institute for Cancer Research published an exhaustive report on the relationship between diet and cancer. The report entitled "Food, Nutrition and Prevention of Cancer: a Global Perspective" was based on an analysis of over 4,500 research studies pertaining to diet and cancer. The following recommendations emerged:

❐ Eat a plant-based diet and reduce your intake of animal-based foods with saturated fats. Eat a variety of fresh fruits and vegetables, beans, legumes, and unrefined grains.

❐ Eat 400 to 800 grams (15 to 30 ounces) of vegetables and fruits every day. This amounts to about five to seven servings (1 cup raw or $1/2$ cup cooked is considered one serving.)

❐ Eat 600 to 800 grams (20 to 30 ounces) of whole grains, beans, legumes, root vegetables, such as potatoes and parsnips, every day. This amounts to about seven servings ($1/2$ cup cooked is considered one serving).

❐ Limit the consumption of refined sugar and refined carbohydrates, like white bread, pasta, and rice.

These recommendations are consistent with those of the American Cancer Society, the US Department of Agriculture, the US Department of Health and Human Services, and many other governmental health agencies, as well as the dietary habits of the healthiest populations on the planet, and, of course, this book.

Wouldn't you agree that it is a better idea to base your decision regarding what to eat on volumes of research, rather than on a few isolated studies pieced together by a fad-diet doctor? Considering the stakes are high—your life is at risk—I'm confident you'd rather base your well-being and the well-being of your family on the former.

A Bushel of Reasons to Eat Carbs

"Let your food be your medicine and your medicine be your food." Hippocrates' words are even more important today than they were 3,000 years ago. Scientists are just now beginning to uncover the medicinal properties of food. Can you imagine a medicine that is able to destroy cancer cells before they get a foothold inside your body, protect normal cells from DNA damage, restructure a cancer cell into a normal healthy cell, and destroy tumors before they have a chance to get started? Can you further imagine that the same medicine can dissolve blood clots before they cause a heart attack or stroke, sweep the bad fat from arteries, and reduce blood pressure to the level it was when you were back in college? All with zero harmful side effects? If a medication like this was available on the market today, drug manufacturers would make a billion dollars overnight. But did you know that you could get all of these benefits and more, simply by eating carbohydrates from heaven?

Researchers are now confirming what mom told us all along—eat your beans, greens, and grains. Scientists have found a special group of substances called *phytochemicals* that are locked inside whole grains, beans, nuts, fruits, and vegetables, and are capable of preventing and reversing diseases. *Phyto* is the Greek word for plant (not Fido, the wonder dog). A mountain of scientific evidence suggests these chemicals found in edible plants are the biggest breakthrough in nutrition since the discovery of vitamins and minerals. White bread, white flour, white rice, and other counterfeit carbs do not provide the health-promoting benefits of the phytochemicals found in carbs from heaven.

But be aware . . . although fresh fruits and vegetables sold in supermarkets may look good, they are likely to be missing many of the life-giving phytochemicals. Conventional produce is typically grown in poor soil, picked before it is ripe, transported across the country, and kept in cold storage. By the time it reaches supermarket shelves, a significant portion of its phytochemicals have been lost. This does not mean that you should pass by the produce; but it does suggest that you try buying local, organically grown varieties whenever possible.

Nature has assembled an entire shopping list of phytochemicals that work together as a team to provide protection against cancer and other chronic diseases. Initial research studies were focused entirely on the health benefits of the fiber found inside unrefined carbohydrates. Now, however, it is understood that fiber, vitamins, minerals, antioxidants, and phytochemicals packaged within whole grains, beans, and legumes all play an important role in protection against cancer.

Nature's Secret Weapon Against Disease

Researchers and clinicians worldwide are proving that phytochemicals can boost the immune system to fight cancer, infections, and many age-related diseases; strengthen the blood vessels to prevent plaguing of the arteries and subsequent heart attacks and strokes; increase blood flow to the brain; increase joint flexibility, improve prostate function; alleviate depression; and increase the ability to cope with stress.

Scientists are astonished that phytochemicals can diffuse cancer cells just like a bomb expert diffuses a bomb before it can cause any damage. Some phytochemicals can change cancer cells into normal healthy cells, while others increase the potency of vitamins, or help improve the communication between different cells. Others are potent antioxidants and provide up to fifty times more antioxidant power than vitamin E. Still others increase the activity of enzymes and hormones.

Whole grains are a virtual storehouse of phytochemicals. Over forty studies have demonstrated that individuals who eat whole grains enjoy up to a 40 percent lower risk of mouth, stomach, colon, gall bladder, and ovarian cancers. Whole grains and beans contain *lignans*—phytochemicals that provide strong protection against cancer. Remember, whole grains also contain valuable anti-cancer nutrients like vitamin E and selenium, but up to 80 percent of these nutrients are lost during the refining process.

Soybeans are a concentrated source of a powerful group of cancer-fighting phytochemicals called *isoflavones*. These plant compounds block enzymes that cause cancer cells to grow and divide. Isoflavones also help to increase bone density, minimize bone loss, and lower cholesterol levels.

Scientists are only just beginning to understand the benefits of the phytochemicals found in edible plants—carbohydrates from heaven. "Every vegetable and fruit has a unique profile of phytonutrients exerting beneficial effects on our bodies to prevent disease," says David Heber, M.D., Ph.D., a professor of medicine and public health at UCLA. Scientists believe phytochemicals are more important than vitamins and minerals. The April 25, 1994 cover article in *Newsweek* magazine had this to say about phytochemicals, "Amid all the debate, phytochemicals offer the next hope for a magic pill, one that would go beyond vitamins."

As you can see, by restricting carbs, you are cutting yourself off from the healing properties of phytochemicals. So, don't forget to follow mom's advice and eat

Phytochemicals Found in Carbs from Heaven

Food	Phytochemical	Benefit
Grains and Beans	Sapporins, Isoflavones	Neutralizes cancer-causing enzymes, reduces cholesterol levels.
Soy beans	Genistein, Diadzein	Alters hormones in a positive way, prevents cancers.
Legumes, nuts, seeds	Phytosterol	Prevents cancers, lowers cholesterol levels.
Grains, beans	Lignans	Prevents cancers.
Flaxseeds, soy beans	Alpha-linolenic acid	Prevents cancers.
Carrots, sweet potatoes, and other orange-colored produce	Carotenoids	Prevents cancers and heart disease, boosts the immune system.
Carrots, citrus fruits, tomatoes, berries	Flavonoids	Blocks cancer-causing hormones, protects and strengthens blood vessels.
Rosemary	Quinone	Neutralizes cancer toxins.
Caraway seeds, mint, basil	Monoterpenes	Antioxidant, potentiates enzymes.

your beans, greens, and grains—and, of course, those fruits and vegetables. Oh, and be sure to show mom the table above, which lists the beneficial phytochemicals found in carbs from heaven. She'll be glad to know she was right all along.

Fiber

A large body of research clearly demonstrates fiber's beneficial role in preventing several types of cancer. Both population studies and clinical studies have shown that fiber, which is found only in carbohydrates from heaven, provides a powerful punch against a wide range of cancers. One study compared the breast cancer rate of women in China (Shanghai and Tianjin) with women in the United States. The

Chinese women had an 80 percent lower breast-cancer rate than the Americans. Out of the 834 women who participated in this study, those who ate the most fiber and the least amount of animal fat, had the smallest incidence of breast cancer. In fact, the women who ate the high-fiber diet had a three times smaller risk of developing breast cancer than the women who ate a low-fiber, high-fat diet.

Phytic Acid (Ip6 factor)

Tucked inside the fiber of cereal grasses and legumes is another carbohydrate called *phytic acid*—also known as the *Ip6 factor*. Recently, scientists have discovered that the Ip6 factor can literally turn off the switch that gives cancer cells the power to grow and divide, while allowing the continued growth of healthy cells.

Dr. A. Shamsuddin, a research scientist at the University of Maryland, and his colleagues, found that the Ip6 factor can literally change a cancer cell back to a normal, healthy cell. Through both animal and human studies, they confirmed that the Ip6 factor packs a powerful wallop against leukemia, cancers of the breast, prostate, lung, liver, and brain. The Ip6 factor strengthens the immune system, helps repair damaged liver cells, has potent antioxidant properties, lowers cholesterol, and prevents kidney stones.

The Ip6 factor is found in all grains, seeds, and nuts. The richest sources by weight include sesame seeds (5.4 percent), lima beans (2.5 percent), soybeans (1.4 percent), corn (1.1 percent), barley (1 percent), whole wheat (0.9 percent), and brown rice (0.9 percent).

> *Considering the anti-cancer properties of Ip6 factor, and all of the other phytochemicals found in carbohydrates from heaven, it is quite obvious that anyone restricting these foods from his diet is stabbing himself in the back.*

How to Make Carbs from Hell "Whole-ier"

Nobody's perfect. You're probably going to eat some carbs from hell from time to time. If you do so only once in a while and still maintain a healthy eating strategy, you can get away with it. But when you do, be sure to follow the simple tips listed below to help you make the bad carbs "better." They will cause less impact on your blood sugar and insulin levels.

Tip 1. When indulging in a carb from hell, be sure to include some high-fiber food to go along with it. Water-soluble fiber in particular slows down the emptying of the stomach contents and the uptake of sugar into the blood. Foods that are high in water-soluble fiber include apples, bananas, pears, oats, barley, beans, legumes, and nuts.

Tip 2. When eating carbs from hell, include several carbs from heaven during the same meal. For example, if you decide you're going to treat yourself to a piece of chocolate-raspberry torte for dessert, plan your meal wisely. For your main meal, for instance, have a bowl of bean soup, a salad, and a baked potato (and be sure to eat the skin).

Tip 3. Scientists have demonstrated that a salad with vinegar helps slow down the absorption of carbs from hell. The acid content in just one tablespoon of vinegar with a meal can lower blood sugar levels by as much as 30 percent. It also helps slow down the emptying of the stomach and the digestion of carbs. Red wine vinegar works best—but lemon, balsamic, apple cider, or rice vinegar all provide the same positive effects.

Tip 4. Exercise can help burn some of the calories from carbs from hell. It also helps maintain blood sugar and insulin levels within normal limits.

Once again, keeping these tips in mind during those times when you indulge in carbs from hell, will help minimize their negative effects.

Summing It Up

Carbs from heaven are certainly among the most impressive of Mother Nature's gifts. In addition to their scientifically proven role in the fight against such conditions as obesity, diabetes, and high blood pressure, this chapter has detailed their amazing role in the prevention of heart disease and cancer. Further proof of their worth is presented in the next chapter, which compares some of the best and worst of the world's most popular diets.

Chapter Eight

Diets of the World
The Good, the Bad, and the Ugly

In 1992, The United States Department of Agriculture (USDA) replaced the out-dated four basic food groups with the USDA Food Guide Pyramid. This "nutri-tion bible," used by dieticians, dieters, and school lunch programs, is even plastered on the back of some bread labels. One of the main recommendations of this pyramid is to eat more carbohydrates and less fat. But there's a problem. The experts who designed this graphic failed to distinguish between good and bad car-bohydrates, and good and bad fats—a big mistake.

The food industry jumped on the government's ill-sighted recommendations and created a multibillion-dollar fat-free market. In no time at all, the buzzwords "fat makes you fat" spread across the country. Americans were given the green light to fill their shopping carts with carbohydrates from hell—the food industry jumped for joy. White bread, white pasta, and desserts laced with white sugar became standard American fare. Consequently, almost overnight, millions of Americans became overweight at an alarming rate

Since its very inception, the USDA Food Guide Pyramid has been criticized by many leading health authorities. According to Dr. Walter Willett, chairmen of the department of nutrition at Harvard School of Public Health, the government's food pyramid isn't doing Americans' expanding waistlines, nor their well-being, any favors. He has also said, "At best, the USDA pyramid offers wishy-washy, sci-entifically unfounded advice on an absolutely vital topic—what we eat," and "At worst, the misinformation it offers contributes to obesity, poor health and unnec-essary early deaths. In either case, it stands as a missed opportunity to improve the health of millions of people." In other words, Dr. Willett believes the USDA Food Guide Pyramid is doing more harm than good.

The government's food pyramid was developed under the direction of the US Department of Agriculture—the agency that promotes the country's agribusiness.

It's obvious that it wasn't developed by an agency that checks and protects public health and well-being. Dr. Willett puts it this way, "Serving two masters is tricky business, especially when one of them includes persuasive and well-connected representatives of the formidable meat, dairy and sugar industries."

The American public has been victimized. The current epidemic of obesity, arthritis, diabetes, heart disease, cancer, and other degenerative diseases is mind-boggling. The stakes are high in the battle of the bulge and chronic degenerative diseases. It's no wonder that health experts and health consumers alike are scratching their heads, groping for dietary guidelines to solve the riddle of illness.

"Old Ways" Provide New Ideas for Americans

Sometimes, the best way to make progress is to return to the past. That is exactly what Oldways International—a high-powered, Boston-based think tank—suggests we should do to solve our modern-day health-care problems. Oldways proposes that we return to traditional diets to dismantle the diseases associated with industrialized nations. The primary goal of its educational programs is to help improve the current dietary guidelines of the USDA and the degenerating health of industrialized nations.

In a joint venture with the Harvard School of Public Health and the World Health Organization (WHO), Oldways has created several diet pyramids that reflect the eating patterns of various cultures from different regions of the world—regions that enjoy exceptional health. These healthy populations were determined through worldwide clinical and epidemiological research, which concluded that a primarily plant-based diet (carbohydrate dominant) that is low in animal protein (saturated fat) is the healthiest eating strategy known to man. These food pyramids are distinctly different from the one created by the USDA, which is based on theory, not on traditional diets that have withstood the test of time.

According to Oldways research studies, three cultural models for healthy living have been clearly identified. They are the traditional diets of the Mediterranean region, Asia, and Latin America. These model diets include centuries-old traditional foods that contribute to optimal health; they also provide delightful tastes and a sense of pleasure—important considerations for everyone.

We live in a society that believes it is more sophisticated and wiser than its ancestors. The good news is that current research is now looking back at the health lessons we can learn from our rich cultural heritage. Although we are an overfed but undernourished nation, somehow, we have convinced ourselves that we enjoy improved health. We ignore the fact that our nation is crippled and dependent on chemical crutches (drugs). Our sinuses drip like faucets, we belch and burp from stomachs that are bloated with gas, our hearts skip and flutter with irregularity, and we are stressed with anxiety and depression. We rely on pills for all of these ills, and long for a true cure. It appears the way to make progress is to go back to the past.

In the following pages, I will present several food guide pyramids that include both contemporary and traditional diets. In addition to the USDA Food Guide Pyramid, I have included modified versions of the Mediterranean, Asian, and Latin American diets, as well as the trendy Low-Carb, High-Protein diet—the "good," the "bad," and the "ugly." Collectively, they are designed to:

❒ Describe the history, benefits, risks, and facts surrounding the different food guide pyramids.

❒ Illustrate inspired, healthy diet traditions, compared to the less-healthful dietary eating styles that are popular in the United States.

❒ Help clear up the confusion surrounding some of the most popular, low-carb diet recommendations.

❒ Help you make informed decisions about your personal food choices.

Each food guide pyramid provides a visual model to help you understand its particular eating strategy. The wide base includes the food(s) with the largest recommended daily intake. Accordingly, as you move up the pyramid, the foods are recommended in lesser quantities. The foods found at the top are to be eaten sparingly.

As you view the traditional diet pyramids of Latin America, the Mediterranean, and Asia, pay particular attention to the position of fruits, vegetables, grains, beans, and meat. In contrast, look at the position of these same foods on the Low-Carb, High-Protein Pyramid. As you will quickly discover, the Low-Carb, High-Protein Pyramid has turned the three traditional diets upside down. Research has demonstrated that by following a low-carb diet, you will be doing the same thing to your health—turning it upside down.

Although the traditional diets of the Latin American, Mediterranean, and Asian people were developed out of necessity and availability, they are a tribute to the creativity of humans. Over time, the people of these regions have transformed simple natural foods into savory gourmet meals, while enjoying lifetimes of good health.

The Fast-Food American Diet

In 1992, the USDA developed the food guide pyramid in an attempt to reduce the country's skyrocketing incidence of diabetes, heart disease, and cancer. But without a time-proven cultural foundation of healthy eating habits to build it on, the creators of this model were forced to base it on educated guesses and corporate influences.

The pyramid's biggest drawback is that it was never tested on an entire population over an extended period of time. Recently, USDA officials have admitted to its failure. In the very near future, the USDA is planning to reveal a new model that actually reflects several of the principles in this book. However, food lobbying groups will undoubtedly try to limit some of these changes.

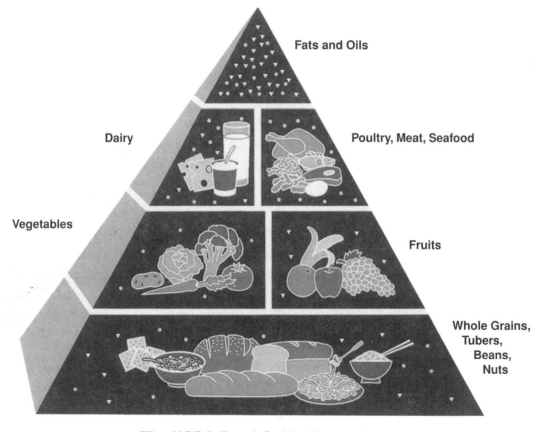

The USDA Food Guide Pyramid
A Dinosaur Heading for Extinction

Facts: The USDA Food Guide Pyramid was designed as a visual aid to encourage Americans to eat a balanced diet of fruits, vegetables, grains, meat, and dairy foods. It encourages carbohydrates to be consumed without guilt, and fats to be consumed with caution. The problem is that it doesn't limit your intake of carbohydrates from hell or encourage you to eat healthy essential fats. But it does increase your risk for health problems, including weight gain, diabetes, heart disease, and cancer.

Carbohydrates: Carbohydrates are at the base of the USDA pyramid. It is suggested that we eat six to eleven servings of cereal, bread, rice, and pasta per day. However this recommendation fails to distinguish between whole grains and refined grains—good and bad carbohydrates. According to the pyramid, all carbohydrates are created equal. Brown rice, white pasta, and Hostess Twinkies are all acceptable and interchangeable sources of carbohydrates.

Although proponents of the USDA food pyramid may state that whole grains are the best choice, very few health care providers pay attention to this recommendation, or give practical advice on how to incorporate them into the diet. Furthermore, even if people wanted to follow this dietary advice, whole grains and unrefined carbohydrates are difficult to find in the American food supply. The bottom line is that the user gets the message that it doesn't make a difference if the carbohydrates are refined or unrefined—because in the end, both types turn into calories.

To its credit, the pyramid places a great deal of emphasis on fruits and vegetables, recommending seven to nine servings per day. Unfortunately, the reality is that less than 10 percent of the adult population follows this advice.

Protein: The USDA pyramid lumps red meat, chicken, turkey, fish, eggs, beans, and nuts together in the protein category. It fails to explain the advantages of plant protein over animal protein, and suggests that all protein foods are equal exchanges and interchangeable. This means that two to three servings of beans, nuts, or fish have the same value as two to three servings of red meat. Yet red meat is high in saturated fat and cholesterol, contains no fiber, and is low in protective antioxidants. On the other hand, nuts and beans are high in beneficial fiber, vitamins, antioxidants, phytonutrients, and unsaturated fats. And fish is low in saturated fat and cholesterol, and an excellent source of omega-3 fats.

Dairy: The pyramid implies that dairy foods are essential and the best source of calcium, recommending two to three servings per day. This leads us to believe that enough dairy products can prevent bone loss and osteoporosis. Ironically, even though the United States is one of the biggest consumers of dairy products in the world, it also has one of the world's highest incidence of osteoporosis.

To further complicate the issue, there is a significant body of research that demonstrates dairy products are linked to many short- and long-term health problems. Acute conditions like recurring ear, nose, throat, bronchial, and bladder infections, and digestive problems like bloating and gas, are all associated with milk allergies. Chronic problems, such as muscle and joint pains, fatigue, constipation, asthma, migraine headaches, and diabetes are also linked to milk allergies. Even some types of cancer, like ovarian and prostate, have been linked to excess dairy consumption.

Better choices of calcium are found in broccoli, Swiss chard, kale, almonds, tofu, and soy milk. A calcium supplement is also a less expensive and healthier source of calcium than dairy products.

Fat: At the top of the USDA pyramid are fats, which we are warned to use sparingly. The problem is that there are good fats and bad fats. Scientists have known since the 1960s that monounsaturated fats (olive oil, walnuts, etc.) and unrefined unsaturated fats (vegetable oils, and oils from fish, nuts, and whole grains) are heart healthy. Yet Americans have been told to curb their intake of all fats. Similarly, since the 1960s, scientists have known that saturated fats found in red meat, poultry, and dairy products, as well as trans fats, also known as hydrogenated oils, promote the artery-clogging process known as arteriosclerosis. This accumulation of arterial plaque leads to heart disease and strokes.

> *The USDA Food Guide Pyramid's biggest drawback is that it was never tested on an entire population over an extended period of time. Recently, USDA officials have admitted its failure.*

Research: Many scholars have suggested that the USDA pyramid is a carefully selected combination of documented research, educated guesses, and economic and politically manipulated information that is closely tied to the meat, dairy, and sugar industries. Critics point out the pyramid provides outdated and misleading information that ignores important research on fats, carbohydrates, and proteins.

Benefits: The USDA food pyramid is a quantum leap forward from the Four Basic Food Groups, which was introduced in 1956 and advised eating a vague "balanced" amount of protein, dairy products, grains, and produce. The newer pyramid provides a much clearer understanding of the amount of food we should eat from each food group and encourages the consumption of more fruits and vegetables.

Risks: Americans have been led to believe that the information provided in the USDA pyramid is a rock-solid guide to good health. But they are being misled. Critics of the guide explain that the government's recommendations are too vague and do not go far enough in explaining the difference between good and bad carbs, plant and animal protein, and good and bad fats. These inadequacies have guided the American public into becoming an overweight population that is riddled with disease.

Present Day: Many of the recommendations found in the USDA Food Guide Pyramid are to blame for our nation's love affair with fast food and its poor nutritional habits. They lead people to believe that a fast food burger and fries are acceptable, and can fulfill part of the daily requirements for carbohydrates, protein, and fat. Such mistaken nutritional information is creating a new generation that eats fewer fresh fruits and vegetables and more burgers, greasy fries, and sugary soft drinks.

A recent study conducted by the National Health and Nutrition Examination Survey tracked the eating patterns of over 15,000 Americans. It concluded that 27 percent of the calories we eat come from fast foods. The study also found that one-third of Americans get 45 percent of their calories from junk food.

If we don't eat healthy, how can we expect our children to? What message are we giving them? What kind of cultural heritage are we leaving for future generations? And who should we blame for the current epidemic of child obesity, diabetes, and heart disease? It should not shock us to hear that our children get a whopping 30 percent of their vegetable requirements from French fries and potato chips. After all, the government's food pyramid considers potato chips and fries "vegetables."

Junk food has become a symbol of America. Two thousand years from now, when archeologists dig up our remains, and they find parts of golden arches, aluminum soda pop cans, potato chip bags, and candy wrappers, it won't take them long to figure out why our civilization was destroyed.

The Color-Soaked Latin American Diet

A group of over 200 scientists, nutritionists, dieticians, chefs, and food journalists constructed the Latin American Food Pyramid. It reflects the culinary traditions of the people from northwestern Mexico to the southern tip of South America and across the Caribbean. The pyramid takes into consideration the wide range of ethnic backgrounds, as well as the educational, economic, and social conditions of the over half-billion people who live south of our nation's border. It also represents the influence of the indigenous Aztecs and Mayan people, as well as the Spanish conquistadors.

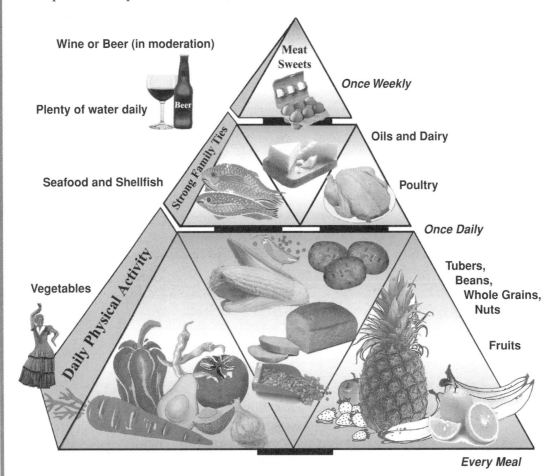

The Latin American Food Pyramid
"You Put the Lime in the Coconut"

Facts: The heart-healthy traditional Latin American diet is built on a framework of carbs from heaven, like fresh fruits and vegetables, beans, potatoes, nuts, chili peppers, and corn. An occasional addition of fish, poultry, and cheese is included. Red meats, eggs, and cheese are eaten sparingly.

Carbohydrates: The indigenous people of Latin America include the Aztecs, Mayans, and Incans. These people relied heavily on carbohydrates like potatoes, sweet potatoes, peanuts, and dried beans, as well as grains, such as quinoa, amaranth, and maize (corn). They consumed these staples two to three times a day, and supplemented them with foods like pumpkin, cassava, squash, papaya, guava, tomatoes, chili peppers, avocados, and pineapples. Honey was their primary sweetener.

These Latin American natives originally ate a primarily vegetarian diet, with a small amount of fish and turkey. The Spanish conquerors introduced cattle, pigs, chickens, dairy foods, oils, sugar, and alcohol—foods and beverages formerly unknown to the natives. They also introduced rice, sugar, bananas, melons, onions, cabbages, and cauliflower.

Protein: Beans, legumes, nuts, corn, and wheat are the primary protein foods included in the Latin American Food Pyramid. At least one of these carbohydrates from heaven is consumed at every meal. Secondary sources of protein foods include fish, eggs, poultry, and red meat. Fish, poultry, eggs, milk, and cheese are eaten in small quantities and only once or twice a week. Red meat is eaten less often — about once a month.

Fat: Vegetable oils are eaten sparingly in the Latin American diet. Greater sources of fat come from nuts, avocados, grains, and vegetables. Fish provides heart-healthy essential fats, while eggs, poultry, milk, cheese, and red meat all provide a small amount of saturated fat.

Research: Epidemiological and clinical studies demonstrate that Latin Americans who adhere to their traditional diets have a lower incidence of heart disease, cancer, and other chronic diseases and conditions associated with the North American diet and lifestyle. Sitting at the foundation of the Latin American Food Pyramid is daily physical activity. The research supporting this pyramid indicates that the level of physical activity promotes weight loss and a high level of wellness.

Benefits: Our friends from the Caribbean and those who live South of the Border who eat their traditional diets are long-lived and healthy populations. They have one of the world's lowest incidences of cancer and other degenerative diseases, and one of the highest life expectancies.

Risks: None. But because the traditional Latin American diet includes small amounts of wine or beer, a word of caution is necessary. Anyone with a history of alcoholism should avoid these beverages.

Present Day: The Americanized version of the Latin American diet bears little resemblance to its "traditional" cuisine. Enchiladas stuffed with beef and smothered under a blanket of cheese and sour cream, along with refried beans made with lard are a typical American interpretation of a much simpler traditional Latin American diet.

The traditional diet of Latin America is still observed by some of the rural populations. Those with sufficient food supplies who eat this traditional diet have low rates of chronic degenerative diseases. However, over the last several decades, as more people have moved to urban areas, many have shifted from their plant-based diets to a high-fat, westernized way of eating.

The people of Latin America who have adopted the dietary habits of western civilizations are now becoming plagued with the chronic diseases associated with "progress." Countries that at one time had to address only the diseases associated with scarcity and starvation, are now facing diseases of affluence, such as obesity, diabetes, and heart disease. For example, obesity and its associated diseases now affect 25 to 50 percent of the people of Mexico. This statistic is not surprising, since average urban dwellers eat a much larger amount of saturated and hydrogenated fat, and sugary, refined carbohydrates from hell than their rural neighbors. They also eat much smaller amounts of fruits and vegetables, and much higher amounts of animal products.

The Pima paradox, which was discussed in Chapter 6, illustrates the adverse effects of a large population group that has abandoned its time-proven traditional Latin American diet. As explained earlier, some of the Pima Indians left Mexico and relocated to Arizona, where they soon abandoned their traditional diet and adopted a high-fat, refined-carbohydrate diet instead. Soon, they were plagued with health problems like obesity, diabetes, and heart disease, although their genetically similar relatives in Mexico, who continued to eat a traditional diet, were virtually free from these diseases. In other words, when the Pima Indians of Arizona began eating large amounts of saturated fat, white bread, white sugar, white rice, and other carbs from hell, they also acquired white man's diseases.

The Adventurous and Delicious Asian Diet

The continent of Asia spans an enormous mass of land that represents a wide variety of people, cultures, and dietary traditions. Oldways International constructed the Asian Food Pyramid in conjunction with Cornell University and the Harvard School of Public Health. The inspiration for the pyramid was drawn from the cuisines of China, Japan, Vietnam, Cambodia, Thailand, Malaysia, Indonesia, Korea, the Philippines, and the other areas of the Pacific Rim.

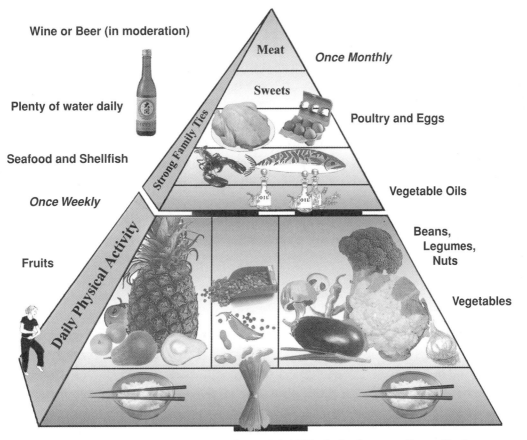

The Asian Food Pyramid
A Time-Honored Tradition

Facts: Carbohydrates form the foundation of the Asian food pyramid. Plant foods, such as noodles, bread, rice, corn, millet, soy beans, mung beans, and other beans and grains, are consumed daily. The next tier of the pyramid includes fruits and vegetables, which are also eaten daily. Nuts are a staple in the Asian diet and an important source of plant protein and essential oils. Dairy foods are almost nonexistent, except in India. Sweets, poultry, and eggs are eaten approximately once a week. Red meat is generally consumed one time per month, or added sparingly to vegetable dishes as a condiment. Green and oolong tea, high in powerful antioxidants, are drunk at meals and believed to contribute to the health and long life of the Asian people. Physical activity, close family relationships, and the pleasure of eating foods with family and friends are other factors that contribute to their good health and longevity.

Carbohydrates: Asians are another major population group that can knock the bottom right out of the low-carb, high-protein diet theory that claims carbohydrates are the cause of weight gain. Rice, a carbohydrate, provides 25 to 75 percent of the total caloric intake of the 2.7 billion people of Asia. This population eats approximately 20 percent more calories (almost entirely from carbohydrates) than the average person living in the United States, yet Americans are 25 percent fatter.

Low-carb diet doctors may have accurately criticized the USDA Food Guide Pyramid recommendations; however, they cannot argue with the time-proven success of the high-carbohydrate, low-protein traditional diet of the Asian population.

Protein: The primary sources of protein in the traditional Asian diet—nuts, beans, and legumes—are used in soups, salads, and main courses. Secondary protein sources, which are used sparingly, include fish, poultry, eggs, and red meat.

Fat: The Asian diet is much like the Mediterranean diet except that it incorporates much less liquid vegetable oil in food preparation. Daily fat intake varies from 8 to 28 percent, but averages about 15 percent of the total calories. Most fat in the Asian diet comes from nuts, seeds, and grains. A small percentage comes from fish, poultry, and red meat.

Research: Scientists have found that the Asian population has one of the lowest rates of degenerative diseases in the world. For example, the death rate from heart disease among the Chinese is seventeen times lower than it is for Americans. Do you think it may be because the Chinese eat approximately three times more fiber? As discussed earlier in this book, fiber is responsible for lowering cholesterol levels and the risk for heart disease. Cholesterol levels of the Chinese people are exceptionally low compared to those of the average American adult. The colon cancer rate for both men and women in China is three times lower than the rate in United States. In Japan, the breast cancer rate is four times lower than that in the United States. It is also interesting that Japanese woman rarely experience menopause symptoms. In fact, there is not a word in the Japanese language to describe menopause.

Scientists in Japan and Switzerland have found that both green tea and oolong tea increase the body's metabolic rate and stimulate weight loss. Drinking between two-and-a-half to five cups of either of these teas per day can burn as much as 80 calories daily. That's about 30,000 calories in one year—or eight-and-a-half pounds.

Benefits: A long life, and protection from heart disease and cancer.

Risks: None. But because the traditional Asian diet includes small amounts of wine or beer, a word of caution is necessary. Anyone with a history of alcoholism should avoid these beverages.

Present Day: The connection between diet and disease is clearly demonstrated in Asian-American immigrants and Asian mainland residents who adopt a westernized diet and lifestyle. Diabetes, osteoporosis, heart disease, and cancer rates have increased dramatically in those individuals who have abandoned their traditional diets and lifestyles.

Surprisingly, scientists have found the incidence of osteoporosis exceptionally low in Asia, despite the fact that dairy products are generally absent from the traditional diet. On the other hand, American eat generous amounts of dairy products, yet have one of the highest rates of osteoporosis worldwide. Asians acquire their calcium from dark leafy green vegetables like broccoli, spinach, and romaine lettuce, as well as almonds and sesame seeds.

Despite documented evidence of the low incidence of osteoporosis in Asians, dairy industry leaders continue to manipulate research to serve their vested interests. Recently, I found an article in the National Dairy Council newsletter entitled, "Milk Helps Put the Brakes on Brittle Bones of Asian Women." The article states, "The Asian diet, typically low in calcium, increases the risk of brittle bone disease (osteoporosis). New research demonstrates that adding milk to the diets of Asian women may be an effective strategy to help halt height and bone loss."

To the casual reader of this article, it would appear that the low calcium intake of the Asian population puts these women at a high risk for brittle bones. That may be true for those Asian women who eat the standard American diet. But the truth is quite the opposite for the women who eat their traditional regional diet. Dr. Colin Campbell of Cornell University, and co-chairperson of the Cornell-China Oxford Project—a massive nutrition and disease study of over 10,000 families living in mainland China—shed light on this subject. According to Dr. Campbell, "The plant-based, dairy-free diet of much of Asia is linked to a low incidence of osteoporosis." The National Dairy Council would like you to believe otherwise.

Dr. Campbell and the experts of the China study concluded that plant-based diets of the Asian population also lowers the rate of heart disease, various cancers, and other diseases associated with industrialized nations. For instance, prostate cancer is the second-leading cause of death in men in the United States. It occurs in 53.4 percent of the country's men, compared to only 1.8 percent of men in Asia. Dr. Campbell's research suggests that replacing animal-based diets with plant-based diets could reduce all cancer in the United States by up to 90 percent.

Green tea and oolong tea, high in powerful antioxidants, are believed to contribute to the health and long life of the Asian people. Regular physical activity, close family relationships, and the pleasure of eating healthful foods with family and friends are other contributing factors.

Another long-term study, the twenty-five year Okinawa Centenarian Study, sponsored by the Japanese Ministry of Health, revealed that the plant-based low-fat diet and lifestyle of the Okinawans is responsible for the healthiest and longest lived population in the world. In fact, the people of Okinawa have the lowest incidence of heart disease, stroke, and cancer in the world. According to the report, "If Americans lived more like the Okinawans, 80 percent of the nation's coronary care units, one-third of the cancer wards, and lots of nursing homes would be shut down."

The Sun-Drenched Mediterranean Diet

The culinary traditions of the Mediterranean region are part of a heritage that turned a diet of necessity into a healthful lifestyle of goodness and pleasure. Created by Oldways International, the Mediterranean Food Pyramid is based on the traditional diets found on the island of Crete, much of mainland Greece, and southern Italy. Variations of the diet are also found in other regions of Italy, France, Spain, Portugal, the Middle East, and parts of Northern Africa.

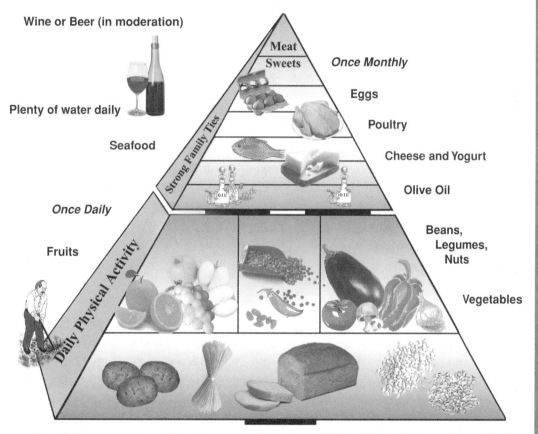

The Mediterranean Food Pyramid
Heart-Healthy and Mouth-Watering

The Facts: The traditional Mediterranean lifestyle goes beyond a beneficial plant-based diet. Typically, the people of the region also lead an inspiring physically active lifestyle and have strong family ties. The region's diet grew out of necessity and availability. Compensating for the lack of meat, the people of the Mediterranean have almost intuitively known how to turn foods like potatoes, whole grains, bread, fruits, vegetables, fresh herbs, beans, legumes, nuts, and seeds into dishes that are both healthy and delicious at the same time.

Secondary to its plant-based mainstays, the Mediterranean diet places fish ahead of eggs, chicken, and red meat. Fish is eaten two to three times per week, chicken is eaten approximately once a week, and red meat is eaten about once a month.

Although the consumption of dairy products is small, very few bone fractures occur among the people of the region. The primary dietary fat comes from extra-virgin olive oil (up to 3 to 4 ounces per day). Wine is generally consumed in small quantities with meals.

Carbohydrates: Carbohydrates are the cornerstone of the Mediterranean diet. The average person living in the Mediterranean region, at least until World War II, grew up on a diet comprised mostly of carbohydrates from heaven—whole grain foods like pasta, rice, cracked wheat, cornmeal, nuts, beans, legumes, fruits, and vegetables, which are all chock full of vitamins, antioxidants, carotenoids, and disease-fighting phytochemicals. Every meal includes fruits, vegetables, beans, and grains. The combination of these ingredients has given birth to a rich and imaginative dietary tradition.

Protein: The Mediterranean diet relies heavily on protein from plant sources, like nuts, beans, and whole grains; however, some protein comes from fish, poultry, and occasionally red meat.

Dairy Products: Most commonly, dairy products are in the form of yogurt or cheese and made from goat and sheep milk, which are very close in chemical composition to mother's milk. They are easily digestible and generally an allergy-free source of dense nutrients. Romano, feta, manchego, and several other delicious cheese varieties made from goat or sheep milk add a wonderful touch to many Mediterranean dishes.

Fat: The principal source of fat in the Mediterranean diet is olive oil—a monounsaturated fat that is high in antioxidants and disease-fighting compounds. Generous amounts of olive oil in the diet are associated with decreased rates of obesity, heart disease, and cancers of the the breast, lung, colon, and skin. The olive oil, nuts, seeds, and fish of the Mediterranean diet provide essential fats that help reduce inflammation and satisfy hunger longer to help maintain good health and normal weight.

Benefits: The Mediterranean diet has been linked to an increased life expectancy and very low rates of heart disease, cancer, and other degenerative diseases that are common in industrialized nations. During the time period of the Seven Country Study (discussed below), deaths from heart disease were 90 percent lower in the Mediterranean region compared to the rates in the United States.

Risks: None. But because the traditional Mediterranean diet includes small amounts of wine with meals, a word of caution is necessary. Anyone with a history of alcoholism should avoid these beverages.

Research: Several studies have demonstrated the heart-healthy benefits of the Mediterranean diet. One study observed 4,000 patients who had had one heart attack. These individuals were put on the Mediterranean diet and observed for four years. The scientists found a 65 percent lower incidence of deaths from second heart attacks in the patients who were on the Mediterranean diet compared to individuals on the American Heart Association's low-fat "Prudent diet."

Research scientists have discovered that tomatoes, one of the all-star foods in the traditional Mediterranean diet, contain a cancer-bashing phytochemical called *lycopene.* The region's classic combination of tomato and olive oil provides the body with a biologically active and concentrated source of lycopene. Researchers have found that five servings of tomatoes per day (one-half cup of tomato sauce is equal to one serving) can provide significant protection against both breast and prostate cancers. Researchers have also observed that one serving of raw tomatoes per week reduces the risk of prostate and breast cancer by 40 percent

Olive oil also reduces the risk of cancer. Harvard research scientists found that women who consume at least two ounces of olive oil per day lower their risk of breast cancer by up to 25 percent.

There is a great deal of interest in the Mediterranean diet for both the medical community and the general population. During the 1950s and 1960s, two major research projects led to interest in this heart-healthy lifestyle—the Seven Country Study, funded by the Rockefeller Foundation, and the follow-up Lyon Study, which was held in Lyon, France. The results of these projects opened the eyes of the medical community to the powerful connection between diet, lifestyle, and coronary heart disease.

During the time of these combined studies, which spanned five to fifteen years, several thousands of individuals were observed. The Seven Country Study found the people with the lowest rate of heart disease lived on the Greek island of Crete. The United States had the highest rate. One of the striking observations made during the course of the project was that 574 Americans but only 9 Cretans died of heart disease—an incredible 98 percent higher incidence for the American subjects. Without a doubt, the Cretans were doing something right to prevent heart disease. Considering one out of every two Americans dies of heart disease every year, scientists wanted to know why.

The researchers concluded that although the people of the southern Mediterranean (Cretans) lived a physically active lifestyle, it was their diet that made the biggest difference. Interestingly, during the study, the Cretans ate four times as

Fish and Mercury Levels

Many regions of the Mediterranean, Latin America, and Asia rely on fish as a dietary staple. Scientists believe this is part of the reason for the good health experienced in these areas. As a result, doctors in the United States, including those of the American Heart Association, recommend eating seafood frequently. That's the good news. Here's the bad news. Some types of fish have high levels of mercury. Eating them too often can cause an accumulation of mercury in the body, resulting in possible memory loss, depression, nerve damage, and heart disease.

Mercury makes its way into the environment—particularly our waterways—through industrial dumping, coal-burning power plants, incinerators, and natural causes, such as volcanoes and forest fires. Once mercury is in the water, it is eaten by bacteria. Small sea creatures eat the bacteria, and then small fish eat the small sea creatures. Finally, bigger fish eat lots of small fish. With each step up the food chain, the concentration of mercury grows. But you don't have to lose your appetite for seafood. When you go fishing in the supermarket, keep the following in mind:

❏ **Safe to eat frequently** (low mercury levels). Wild salmon, sardines, tallapia, orange roughy, shrimp, scallops, oysters, and "organic" farm-raised salmon.

❏ **Safe to eat occasionally** (moderate mercury levels). Ocean trout, flounder, mahi-mahi, red snapper.

❏ **Avoid or eat rarely** (high mercury levels). Chilean sea bass, shark, swordfish, grouper, halibut, tuna.

many whole grain bread (carbs) as their American counterparts, thirty times more beans and legumes (carbs), six times more fish, three times more fat (mostly olive oil), and twice as many vegetables (carbs). Every main meal included a generous portion of dark leafy green vegetables (carbs).

Two of the most striking statistics that were revealed during the Seven Country Study included the following:

1. The study subjects from the island of Crete ate four times more carbohydrates (bread) than their American counterparts, yet obesity was rare.

2. The Americans in the study consumed eight times more meat than their Cretan counterparts, but the Cretans had 98 percent fewer deaths from heart disease, the number-one killer disease in the American population.

The largest fish, which contain the highest levels of mercury, usually have the least amount of heart-healthy oils. On the other hand, some of the best sources of the heart-healthy omega 3 fats, such as salmon and sardines, have much lower mercury levels.

Conventional farm-raised salmon have very high levels of mercury, and scant amounts of the heart-healthy essential oils. These farm-raised salmon, have low levels of the beneficial omega-3 fats. The problem arises because conventionally farm-raised salmon are fed meat scraps and grains (wild salmon eat sardines and herring). Consequently, instead of having a natural bright orange color and high levels of omega-3 fats, most farm-raised salmon are pale grey and contain small amounts of essential oils. In an effort to get the fish to look more natural, companies inject them with a hazardous orange-colored dye. Not all farmed salmon, however, are raised this way. Some companies raise them organically, which results in fish that retain their natural color and contain high-levels of omega-3 fats.

If you frequently eat large-fish varieties, have yourself tested periodically for mercury levels. A hair analysis is the most accurate test to detect body levels of mercury and other heavy metals, such as lead and aluminum. Hair is a stable tissue that provides a long-term ticker tape of heavy metal accumulation. Red blood cells, which are replaced every ninety days, will not provide long-term information. Laboratories that perform this test normally screen a panel of several heavy metals. Ask your doctor about this test.

It is quite clear from these statistics that good carbs promote a fit and trim body, and help prevent heart disease at the same time. On the other hand, the high saturated-fat content of several popular low-carb diets is the main culprit that promoted the high incidence of heart disease in the above studies.

The Cretans had 98 percent fewer deaths from heart disease, the number-one killer in the American population. Dr. Ansel Keys, the chairperson of this study, commented that heart disease was virtually nonexistent in the Cretan population group—except within a small class of wealthy people who had meat in their diet every day.

Present Day: The results of the Seven Country Study gave rise to some new questions for the scientific community. Could different populations get the same heart-healthy benefits from the Mediterranean diet as those who lived on Crete? Would the Mediterranean diet be as effective as the American Heart Association's (AHA) low-fat Prudent diet, which replaced butter with margarine, beef with chicken, bacon and eggs with cold cereal and toast, whole milk and cream with skim milk, and lard with vegetable oil. And finally, could people living in the westernized world, Americans in particular, get accustomed to the Mediterranean diet?

In the 1990s, scientists conducted a follow-up research study in Lyon, France, to answer these questions. The research group was made up of 605 patients who had recently had a heart attack. These individuals were randomly divided into two groups. The control group was placed on the low-fat Prudent diet, while the second group followed the Mediterranean diet.

After only two months, a significant difference in the overall health of the two groups was observed. At the end of the first year, only 2 percent of the group on the Mediterranean diet had had a second heart attack or stroke, compared to 14 percent of those on the Prudent diet. By the end of the second year, only 4 percent of the Mediterranean diet group had experienced a second heart attack, compared to 19 percent of the group on the Prudent diet. By the end of the third year, the low-fat group saw a whopping 27 percent rise in heart attacks and strokes; the Mediterranean diet group had only 6 percent. The benefits of the Mediterranean diet were obvious.

After three years, those who had been following the Prudent diet switched to the Mediterranean diet, and two years later, the researchers did a follow-up study. The group experienced a 68 percent lower incidence of heart attacks, and 56 percent fewer cases of cancer.

The "High-Risk" Low-Carb, High-Protein Diet

It is ironic that the low-carb, high-protein diet was first popularized by an overweight undertaker named William Banting around 1863. At that time, Banting was under the care of a young physician named William Harvey, who theorized that carbohydrates increased the formation of fat. Banting lost forty-six pounds on Dr. Harvey's low-carb, high-protein diet, and wrote about his experience in a paper that eventually sold over 100,000 copies. Banting's name was actually listed as a verb in the *Concise Oxford Dictionary* until 1963. "To bant" or "banting" was defined as *the treatment of obesity by abstinence from sugar and starch.*

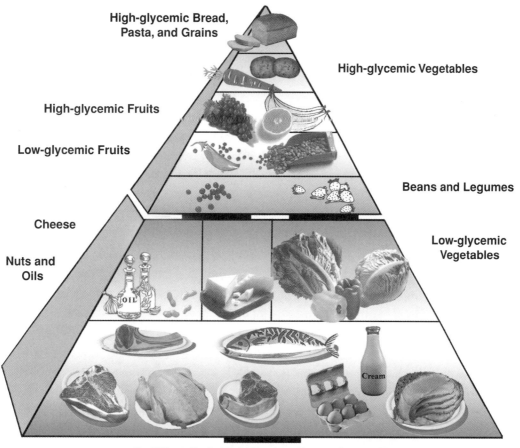

High-glycemic Bread, Pasta, and Grains

High-glycemic Vegetables

High-glycemic Fruits

Low-glycemic Fruits

Beans and Legumes

Cheese

Low-glycemic Vegetables

Nuts and Oils

Red Meat, Pork, Fish, Poultry, Butter, Cream, Eggs

The Low-Carb, High-Protein Food Pyramid

Lose Weight Today . . . Forget About Tomorrow

Although the verb "to bant" died 100 years after Banting first popularized the low-carb diet, Dr. Robert Atkins resurrected the low-carb, high-protein diet in the 1970s with his first book, *Dr. Atkins' Diet Revolution*. Since then, there have been several variations of this diet fad, including the Zone, South Beach, and Stillman diets. Incidentally, Dr. Stillman died of a heart attack. I hope more people learn the "heart- jeopardizing"truth about high-protein, low-carb diets before possibly meeting the same fate.

The Facts: Although the various low-carb diets are slightly different from each other, they all share several common beliefs, spearheaded by the idea that carbohydrates are the villains responsible for weight gain. Several low-carb diet doctors claim that in order to be fit and trim, we must reduce our intake of carbs, while increasing protein and fat. According to some of these weight-loss formulas, instead of adding generous amounts of potatoes, carrots, and whole grain bread to our plates, we are told to eat decadent portions of sausage, steak, and lobster drenched in butter. It's no surprise why this type of diet is so popular in this country—millions of Americans love eating meat and other high-fat foods. It simply tells people what they want to hear.

Staunch carb opponents claim that because carbs raise blood sugar levels, they automatically raise insulin levels and trigger the storage of fat. Additionally, they claim protein and fat do not raise blood sugar levels, and, therefore, do not raise insulin levels. Consequently, the body will burn fat. However, research demonstrates a different picture. For example, beef raises insulin levels 27 percent more than whole grain pasta. The truth is, protein *does* raise blood insulin levels, sometimes even higher than carbohydrates.

Carbohydrates: It is hard to believe, but low-carb diet doctors have convinced millions of confused Americans that sausage is better for you than a baked potato, pork rinds are healthier than carrots, and a hamburger will peel off the weight faster than an apple. However, in their defense, they do wisely suggest that refined sugar, white bread, white rice, and processed convenience foods are the worst possible carbs. Next in line on the low-carb hit list are carbs that quickly raise blood sugar levels—high-glycemic carbs. But as you learned in Chapter 6, the glycemic index is misleading. Consequently, innocent carbs from heaven like carrots and potatoes are banished. The bottom line is that all low-carb diets restrict carbs—some more than others.

Protein: The high-protein content of this diet is detrimental to overall health. Research has proven that high-protein diets cause calcium to be lost through the urine, increasing the risk for bone loss and osteoporosis. High-protein intake also raises uric acid levels in the blood, increasing the chances of gout and kidney stones. Excess dietary protein produces too much acid, one of the main causes of chronic disease according to doctors of alternative medicine.

Fat: Many low-carb, high-protein diets recommend large amounts of animal protein that are high in saturated fat, which scientists have linked to heart disease and several types of cancer (see the charts on pages 146 and 147). Interestingly, a few short-term studies have demonstrated that the Atkins' Diet lowers cholesterol and triglyceride levels. This, however, is not surprising, because whenever there is a reduction in weight, there is an automatic reduction in cholesterol and triglycerides. Dr. James Anderson from the University of Kentucky Metabolic Center, calculated that in the long term, diets high in saturated fat will elevate cholesterol by 28 percent, whereas low-fat diets will decrease it by 21 percent.

Research: Doctors at Duke University Medical School found that test subjects following a high-protein diet for six months, lost an average of twenty pounds. However, a significant number of these patients also displayed a number of disturbing side effects, including constipation, headaches, irritability, hair loss, and bad breath. Critics also warn that low-carb, high-protein diets increase the risk of kidney damage, bone loss, elevated cholesterol, heart disease, and some cancers. By contrast, the patients I put on my high-carb, low-fat American-MediterrAsian diet routinely lose from twenty to thirty pounds in eight to ten weeks—without any short- or long-term health risks. They lose weight without counting calories or "mortgaging" their health in the process.

Benefits: Short-term weight loss.

Risks: Low-carb diets pose a real threat to short- and long-term health. Short-term problems can include headaches, irritability, constipation, bad breath, and dehydration. Long-term problems can include kidney stones, osteoporosis, heart disease, and cancer. They may take years to surface as they slowly erode health before spiraling into serious life-threatening conditions or diseases. Many physicians, researchers, and government health agencies are warning people of these dangers.

Present Day: Although first introduced in the 1970s, the Atkins' Diet gained a surge of recent interest and has become one of the most popular low-carb, high-protein diets in the nation. In 2002, Dr. Atkins' *New Diet Revolution* made this diet seem like the latest scientific breakthrough, leading people to believe it would change the history of weight loss. Yet, the Atkins' Diet and other versions of the low-carb diet craze have merely resurrected a diet that has existed for over 100 years. One must ask the question: If low-carb diets didn't work before, why would anyone think they are going to work now, especially with all of the potential health risks?

A lot of questionable science surrounds Dr. Atkins' theories. People do lose weight on low-carb, high-protein diets—but only temporarily. However, as you have already learned, they are losing it for all the wrong reasons. According to Frederick Samaha, M.D., assistant professor of medicine and chief of cardiology at the Philadelphia Veterans Administration Hospital and lead investigator for the

Breast Cancer & Saturated Fat Consumption

Approximately one out of every ten women die of breast cancer every year. Billions of dollars are spent on surgeries and/or therapies; yet, very little effort is made on educating our meat-hungry nation of the link between saturated fat and breast cancer. Studies have demonstrated the higher the saturated fat in the diet, the greater the risk for breast cancer. As seen in the chart below, the populations with the highest consumption of saturated fat, have the highest incidence of breast cancer.

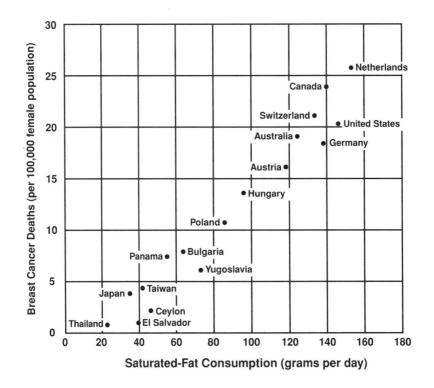

Atkins' Diet study, individuals on this diet did lose more weight than those on a low-fat diet. However, the weight loss resulted from eating fewer calories. (See the low-carb calorie tally on page 93). According to Dr. Samaha's report in *The New England Journal of Medicine*, "The low-carb group was eating, on average, 460 fewer calories per day than when they came into the study, compared to just 270 calories less for the high-carb group."

Do people keep the weight off? Not for long. Most people find it too difficult to maintain this diet as a permanent lifestyle. Keeping off the weight is about as likely

Prostate Cancer & Saturated Fat Consumption

Scientists at Loma Linda University studied the effect of saturated fat on over 6,500 men for one year. They found those who ate the most saturated fat, had almost four times the incidence of prostate cancer. The following chart shows the same pattern in world populations. The populations with the highest saturated-fat intake derived from meat consumption have the highest incidence of prostate cancer.

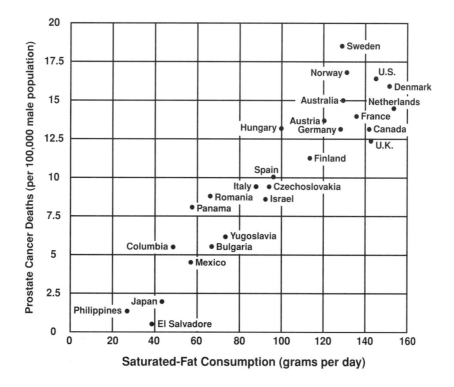

as being the winner of a casino jackpot—it *can* happen, but the odds are against you. There are plenty of short-term success stories of people who have lost weight on low-carb diets, but very few keep it off for the long term. Those who lose weight on low-carb diets almost always end up putting it back on—often with a vengeance.

Still not convinced low-carb diets are a waste of time? Maybe this will finally convince you. Scientists at Brown University and Colorado University have created the National Weight Control Registry—the largest collection of long-term weight-loss testimonies in the world (www.nwc.ws). Any individual who has lost at least thirty pounds and has maintained the loss for more than one year is qualified to register. Although proponents of low-carb diets encourage their participants to register with the database, few, if any, have been able to qualify. In an article in the June 16, 2003, *U.S. News and World Report,* according to Dr. Rena Wing, one of

> *. . . according to Dr. Rena Wing, one of the founders of the National Weight Control Registry, out of over 3,000 people who have already registered with the National Weight Control Registry, "Nobody is maintaining their weight loss with a diet low in carbohydrates." I hope you will think twice before trying a low-carb diet.*

the founders of the National Weight Control Registry, of the over 3,000 people who have already registered, "Nobody is maintaining their weight loss with a diet low in carbohydrates."

I hope you will think twice before trying a low-carb diet. Short-term success stories of low-carb dieters are real; however, the real truth is that long-term weight loss rarely occurs. Over 15 million copies of Dr. Atkins' latest diet book have already been sold. Another 15 million will probably be sold on recycled hype without proof of long-term weight loss or safety—two major considerations.

Under normal circumstances, there isn't a population of people on God's green earth who eat a restricted low-carb diet—with the exception of the Eskimos, who, by the way, have a short life span. In fact, in order to make up for the lack of nutritious fruits, vegetables, and grains in their carbohydrate-scarce diets, Eskimos derive a great deal of their vitamins and minerals by consuming the nutrient-rich organs—eyes, glands, and gonads—of their prey. Could you imagine the average American low-carb diet enthusiast at the dinner table saying, "Please pass the gonads?" Simply put, low-carb diets are not normal eating patterns for humans.

Eskimos eat about 250 to 350 grams of protein per day, which is not an unrealistic amount for someone on a high-protein diet. Eskimos also have the highest incidence of osteoporosis in the world—despite the fact that they consume an average of 2,200 milligrams of calcium per day. And how can low-carb diet doctors explain the Asian population? Asians are one of the thinnest populations on the planet, and yet they eat a high-carbohydrate, low-animal protein diet. (They consume at least 20 percent more carbohydrates than Americans.) In addition to the Asian population, scientists have documented that the people who live in the Mediterranean region and Latin America who follow their traditional high-carb, plant-based diets, have a low incidence of obesity and chronic disease. Go figure.

A Closer Look at a Popular Low-Carb Diet

Dr. Robert Atkins, the grandfather of the low-carb diet doctors, has created the most popular of the low-carb diets. Let's take a closer look.

During the first two weeks of the diet, you are allowed to eat as much protein and fat as you want from foods like steak, sausage, bacon, eggs, cream, and butter. At the same time, you are to restrict carbohydrate intake to 20 grams or less. To give you an idea of how ridiculously low this is—one-third of a bagel is equal to 20 grams of carbohydrates. Bread is out of the question. And you'll also have to ditch the apple because it exceeds the 20-gram limit. Pasta, potatoes, and rice are out of bounds. What's left are only low glycemic-index carbohydrates like salad greens, broccoli, cabbage, and berries.

Once you have reached your desired weight, you can add 5 grams of carbs back into your diet per week, until you reach the point at which you start to gain weight. This is called the "maintenance phase." During this period, you can eat approximately 40 to 90 grams of carbs. The exact amount is determined by the set point at which you started to gain weight. This means, if you made the Atkins' Diet a lifetime plan, at most, you would be allowed about 90 grams of carbohydrates per day (the equivalent of one bagel and an apple). Not a pretty picture is it?

People get excited about this diet because they are able to lose weight quickly while on it, but it has its own set of serious side effects. One is called *ketosis*, an abnormal condition that the Atkins' proponents make sound like a blessing in disguise. When the body does not have enough carbohydrates at it's disposal to produce glucose for fuel, it will resort to burning stored fat and muscle for fuel through the ketosis process. Ketosis is one of the body's last-ditch emergency efforts to make glucose for energy. Through this act of desperation, fat and muscle are broken into ketones. In the process, large amounts of water are lost and appetite is suppressed, causing decreased calorie intake and, therefore, weight loss. In reality, ketosis is a "sick person" condition. Diabetics, pregnant women with toxemia, and starving bodies can all develop it, which, in certain conditions, can even be fatal.

Ketosis is toxic to the body. An outward sign and clue that ketosis is not good for anyone's health is that it causes bad breath. Worse than a dog's breath. But even more serious, ketosis can cause nausea, constipation, headaches, irritability, light-headedness, muscle breakdown, dehydration, and kidney damage. For these reasons alone, why would anyone want to go on such a bizarre diet? One that doesn't amount to anything more than a calorie-restrictive eating plan with some potentially serious short- and long-term adverse health effects.

Dr. Richard M. Fleming is a cardiologist and founder of the Fleming Heart & Health Institute in Omaha, Nebraska. His research showed that after one year, study subjects on the Atkins' Diet developed inflammation in the inner lining of blood vessels and had a 40-percent decrease in blood flow to the heart. Dr. Fleming found that these individuals had high levels of C-Reactive protein—a marker in the blood for inflammation and a predictor of heart disease. He concluded that the Atkins' Diet creates a high risk for heart disease, even in the short run.

Researchers at the University of Texas, Southwestern, conducted a six-week study to determine the effects of a low-carb, high-protein diet on kidney function. The study, reported in the August 2002 *Journal of Kidney Disorders*, revealed what scientists have feared all along—the threat of kidney damage on a low-carb, high-protein diet is real—not theoretical. The study subjects experienced a 55-percent calcium loss in their urine, moving them toward bone loss, kidney stones, and kidney failure.

Dr. Paul Crawford, chairman of the American Kidney Fund and lead investigator of the study said, "We have long suspected that high-protein weight-loss diets could have a negative impact on the kidneys, and now we have research to support our suspicions. Dehydration forces the kidneys to work harder to clean toxins from the blood. The kidneys not only filter the blood, they help regulate blood pressure and the number of red blood cells." Dr. Crawford further explained that high-protein diets lead to the buildup of nitrogen in the urine, which further strains the kidneys. According to Dr. Crawford, "Chronic kidney disease results from hyperfilteration (strain on the kidneys), produces scarring in the kidneys, reducing kidney function." Scarring and reduced kidney function can lead to chronic kidney disease. Dr. Crawford warns that, "Chronic kidney disease is not to be taken lightly and there is no cure for kidney failure."

Interestingly, Dr. Atkins tried to make people believe that ketosis is heaven on earth for anyone who wants to lose weight. But as you can see, ketosis and low-carb, high-protein diets actually put the body through hell. Atkins claimed kidney damage wouldn't result from his diet because ketosis occurs for only a couple weeks; however, he himself warned individuals with kidney disease and those who are pregnant not to go on the diet. Furthermore, the diet suggests that any time a person gains weight, he or she should induce ketosis to stimulate weight loss. Consequently, it is not unusual for people on the Atkins' Diet to bounce in and out of ketosis over and over again, putting undo stress on the kidneys.

The high saturated-fat content in Atkins' and similar low-carb, high-protein diets poses another risk—heart disease. In fact, in 2002, the American Heart Association issued a warning that a high-protein diet not only increases the risk for heart disease, it also increases the risk for strokes, diabetes, and certain types of cancer. Robert Eckel, chairman of the AHA's nutrition committee said, "It is our opinion that as a tool for dealing with 'fat America,' it carries the very real potential for an increased risk of heart attack."

Low-carb diets radically restrict fruits, vegetables, grains, and beans, dramatically reducing intake of the many cancer-protective phytochemicals found in these foods. Dr. Gladys Block of the University of California reviewed over 170 nutrition studies from seventeen countries. She discovered populations that eat the most fruits, vegetables, grains, and beans have 50 percent less incidence of cancer compared to those populations who eat the least amount of these foods.

Another consideration of low-carb, high-protein diets is their wastefulness. According to John Robbins, author of *The Food Revolution*, the United States consumes 23 percent of the world's beef supply, yet makes up only 4 percent of the world's population. The Atkins' Diet more than doubles the intake of meat Americans already eat. This means, in order to sustain this diet, we would need almost 50 percent of the world's supply of beef. Robbins says 40 percent of the world's grain is used to fatten up livestock—grain that could be fed to a hungry world. He also points out that each year it would require 12 million tons of grain to adequately feed all of the starving people on the entire planet. We could free up 12 million tons of grain simply by reducing our intake of meat by a mere 10 percent. On the other hand, just think of how much grain we would use if we increased our meat consumption by 50 percent, as the Atkins' Diet suggests.

Many people think Dr. Atkins was a genius. Many people think he was a fool. I believe he was a good businessman who fashioned a fad diet with an ingenious marketing plan. The truth of the matter is that all low-carb diet doctors are gambling on their unproven theories. The stakes are high—the health of millions of Americans is at risk. Just like the card dealers in a casino, the low-carb diet doctors are relying on their own cleverness. Only instead of money, the lives of millions of desperate, over-weight people are on the table. Even the outcome is the same. Although people do win a little in the short run (temporary weight loss), in the end, the dieter will lose. Instead of bankrupting people's life savings, diet doctors may be bankrupting something more valuable—their victims' health. Are you willing to gamble with yours?

Before you decide to follow a low-carb high protein diet, ask yourself the following question. Are you willing to give up harmless foods like potatoes, bread, pasta, rice, corn, and other innocent carbohydrates based on the unproven theories of a handful of diet doctors? Is it wise to follow these diet gurus who spread grains of truth mixed with misleading advice?

It's Not About Deprivation

The next time you pass by a kitchen, stop and take a whiff. You might notice the heavenly aroma of whole grain bread baking in the oven, or a bowl of piping hot whole wheat pasta smothered in pesto sauce. You might enjoy the tantalizing smell of an apple, cherry, or blueberry pie, sweetened with raw honey and housed in a crisp whole wheat crust. Remember, you don't have to sacrifice these delicious-tasting carbohydrates to win the battle of the bulge. Moderation, not deprivation, of these wholesome foods is the key to a fit and trim body. With carbs from heaven on your plate, the right amount of exercise, and a positive attitude toward a healthy lifestyle, you will not only win the battle of the bulge, you will also gain a lifetime of wellness.

Carbohydrates from heaven are not the cause of obesity—carbohydrates from hell are! Even the Atkins' camp agrees with this statement. According to Colette Heimowitz, Director of Education and Research at the Atkins' Health and Medical Information Services in New York City, "You can succeed on a low-fat diet if you control your calories and choose foods such as fruits, vegetables and whole grains." She concludes her statement by saying, "It's when you add refined carbs to the mix that you run into trouble." Need I say more? I rest my case.

The Choice Is Yours

You can follow the guidelines of the USDA Food Guide Pyramid, with its flawed perspective on carbohydrates and fats, and rigged advice from the meat, dairy, and sugar industries; follow the latest low-carb, high-protein fad diet, with its high risk for unhealthy short- and long-term side effects; or enjoy good taste and good health with the time-proven dietary traditions from the Mediterranean, Latin American, or Asian populations—the healthiest in the world. The choice is yours.

Part 3

Living Well

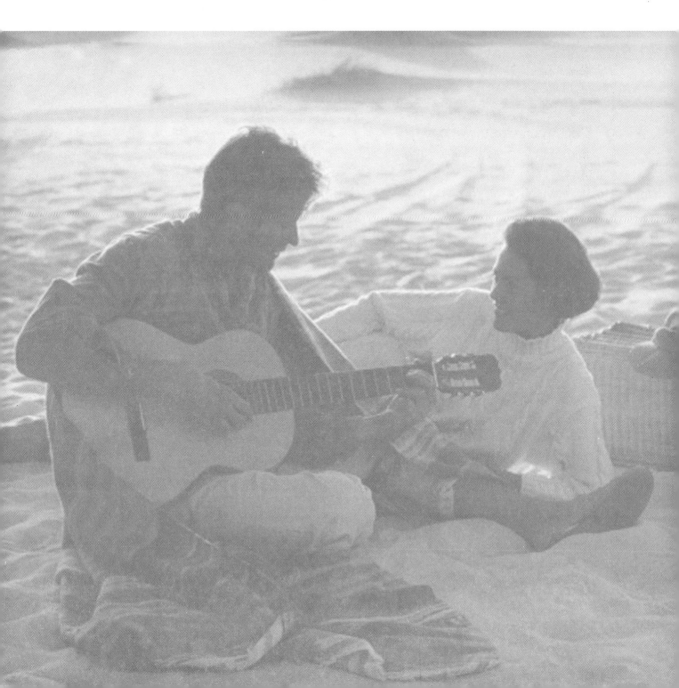

Chapter Nine

Prescription for Wellness

"Those who do not find some time every day for health,
must one day sacrifice a lot of time for illness."

—Father Sebastian Kneipp
19th Century Health Advocate

Would you like more energy, greater enthusiasm, and an increased sense of well-being? Remember, health should be your first goal, not weight loss. Permanent weight loss is the outcome of a healthy lifestyle, not a fad diet. The good news is that all of these health benefits, as well as a trim body, are within your reach, but you must take charge of your own well-being. You are the one who makes the final decisions to improve your health—or run it into the ground. Your doctor can give you advice, but it is you who must make the commitment and take the steps toward wellness. More than likely, you have heard the word "wellness" before. But do you know what it means?

Wellness is not just the mere absence of illness. Rather, it describes a lifestyle that is characterized by optimum physical, emotional, and mental well-being. It is a healthy alternative to a lifetime bent on drugs, surgery, and illness. But wellness must be earned, requiring a commitment to reach your personal health potential. Wellness encourages you to cultivate healthy habits—like eating the right foods, exercising, laughing, forgiving others, taking time for prayer, developing healthy relationships, and keeping a positive mindset. If you have an illness, pursuing wellness will uplift your spirits and encourage a vision of hope and healing. Actively pursuing wellness automatically helps prevent disease. If you have an illness, wellness will help release your body's healing power and reduce symptoms.

Be proactive in achieving quality in your life, not a spectator. There are a number of active steps you can take when traveling the road to wellness. For starters, try to associate with other individuals who also want to achieve wellness. A wellness buddy or coach will support you, and help get you back on your feet if you fall. If you have tried in the past to live a healthier lifestyle, but lost your motivation, don't look back on those attempts as worthless failures—rather consider them stepping stones toward eventual success. Set realistic goals. Be specific, but above all, be patient. Reach your wellness goals by taking it one step at a time. As you add more healthy habits, and eliminate harmful ones, you will gradually tip the scale in the direction of wellness.

Take advantage of modern medicine when you need it, but don't count on it to achieve wellness. Treatment with drugs and surgery has helped save the lives of millions of people, but it also has some serious limitations. We have the world's best emergency health care system. Modern medicine is outstanding in the event of serious infections, traumatic injury, heart attacks, strokes, and other emergencies. But treating nonemergency conditions with drugs and surgery is another story. The resulting side effects can often be worse than the original condition.

Orthodox medicine has only scratched the surface when it comes to the prevention and treatment of diseases associated with aging. How many years have we heard that a cure for cancer, heart disease, diabetes, arthritis, and other serious illnesses are just around the corner? Don't hold your breath! The cures are nowhere in sight. Prevention is the key. A wellness lifestyle is your best insurance policy. If you are fighting a chronic illness, wellness will give your body the power to win the battle.

Whatever condition your health is in right now, you can improve it by making a commitment to wellness. It will help you banish any symptoms you may have been suffering with for months or even years. You will be able to say good riddance to headaches, indigestion, sinus problems, high blood pressure, high cholesterol, constipation, irritable bowel syndrome, chronic coughing, skin rashes, muscle and joint pains, poor concentration, and many other symptoms you may have thought you'd have to live with for the rest of your life!

So how do you say goodbye to illness and hello to wellness? First of all, it is important to recall that most people are born with wellness. The body and mind are at ease, free from *dis-ease*—a term that indicates "lack of ease" or balance. The problem begins when we start to acquire bad habits that disturb our ease. Poor nutrition, inactivity, unmanaged stress, insufficient water intake, smoking, and excessive alcohol consumption are some of these habits. To add insult to injury, we take over-the-counter and prescription medications to cover up the symptoms we acquire from our bad habits. We are also exposed to chemicals in the air we breathe, the water we drink, and the food we eat. Over time, these factors slowly whittle away at our body's state of ease, causing dis-ease.

To eliminate dis-ease and restore ease to your life, you must be willing to take responsibility for your health. By taking charge, you can break free from the trappings of illness and move back into the circle of wellness. The "7 Steps to Living Well" will show you how.

7 Steps to Living Well

The "7 Steps to Living Well" are stepping stones to wellness—easy guidelines for an all-around healthy lifestyle. Steps 1 and 2, presented in this chapter, are designed to help you set the groundwork and start you on the right path. Steps 3 through 5, which focus on eating for good health, are found in Chapter Ten, while final Steps 6 and 7, designed to energize your life, are presented in Chapter Eleven. Make the commitment to wellness, and enjoy the journey.

7 Steps to Living Well

Step 1	Find a Wellness Coach.
Step 2	Track your progress.
Step 3	Eat a rainbow.
Step 4	Balance carbs, protein, and fat.
Step 5	Take advantage of power carbs.
Step 6	Don't work out, get energized.
Step 7	Chuckle every day—to keep the doctor away.

Step 1. Find a Wellness Coach

Could you imagine a baseball player without a coach? An Olympic athlete without a trainer? How about a student without a teacher? Life coaches help us to reach our highest level of achievement. Michael Jordan was a good basketball player—but his coaches helped to make him the best. Without leadership, without discipline or guidance to stretch us beyond our comfort zone, our ability to reach high levels of achievement would diminish.

A wellness coach offers the same advantages. He or she is a motivator who gently moves you out of your comfort zone, provides support, stretches your perception of optimal health, and helps you build the foundation for a lifetime of wellness. A wellness coach shines a light on the weaknesses in your lifestyle, and helps you see your way through health challenges. Leading by example, this person is a mentor who is self-disciplined and physically active—someone who encourages optimal health and well-being. A wellness coach is not perfect; however, he or she is tenacious and has stick-to-itiveness—a role model who helps guide you along the path to wellness.

A wellness coach can be a family member, a friend, a neighbor, or your doctor. Do you know the word "doctor" literally means "teacher"? It's true. The word comes from the Latin word *docere*—which means "to teach." Doctors are supposed to teach patients how to achieve optimal health. They *should* be wellness coaches, leading a healthy lifestyle and setting an example for patients to follow. Doctors *should* encourage patients to take an active role in their heath care. Does your doctor fit this description?

Unfortunately, most doctors today do very little teaching. They are more apt to merely prescribe pills and perform surgery. Very few make good wellness coaches. Most encourage their patients to rely only on their treatments. They tend to diagnose and treat, rather than evaluate and educate. Consequently, most people who visit their doctors are passive recipients rather than active participants in their health care. Don't be a passive recipient. I encourage you to

> *Most doctors encourage their patients to rely only on treatments. They tend to diagnose and treat, rather than evaluate and educate. Consequently, most people who visit their doctors are passive recipients rather than active participants in their health care.*

take charge of your health. If your doctor is not a good wellness-coach candidate , look elsewhere to find one. However, be sure to keep your doctor informed of your lifestyle changes.

Good wellness coaches offer many advantages. They can teach you how take more of an active role in your health care. They can help you pinpoint any day-to-day choices that are interfering with your ability to experience optimal health, and help you develop strategies to overcome those obstacles.

If you have an illness, it would be worthwhile to consult a doctor who is a wellness coach, even if it means traveling a long distance to get to his or her office. Keep in mind that most people with a mild to moderate illness do not need medication—they need education. Develop a partnership with a physician who doesn't have a hyperactive hand—and a prescription pad. Find a doctor who will provide any necessary therapy, as well as healthful strategies for positive lifestyle changes.

If you are already in good health, a wellness coach can help you reach an even higher level, and bolster disease prevention. Remember, your diet and lifestyle can either build and maintain your level of good health—or encourage illness.

Step 2. Track Your Progress

Your first step toward wellness should begin with a personalized wellness plan. Setting short- and long-term goals, and charting your progress on the road to good health will help you to stay on track as you move forward.

What follows are some ideas for possible goals. In the short-term, for example, goals can include changing your wardrobe to improve your appearance, exercising fifteen minutes per day, drinking more water, developing new friendships with others who are on a path to wellness, keeping a diet diary, increasing your intake of whole grains and beans, decreasing your intake of meat, trying new foods with different tastes and textures, reading food labels at the supermarket, replacing over-the-counter medications with natural remedies, and taking a class on stress management. In the long term, you may decide that you want to: lose twenty pounds, work with your doctor to get off prescription drugs, walk two miles a day, train for a marathon race, join a basketball league, or become an aerobics instructor.

When setting goals, keep in mind that "big changes begin with small steps." Once you have decided on the behavior(s) you would like to change, the following guidelines will help keep you on track:

❏ Set a goal and create steps for achieving it. (See the sample progress chart on page 161.) Also document how you and others will be affected by these changes.

❏ Start off on a small scale. Breaking down a major long-term goal into several smaller short-term goals will make your long-term goal seem more do-able. For example, if you want to lose fifty pounds over the course of the next year, your short-term goal may be to lose one pound per week.

❏ Try to keep up with the latest news on health and nutrition, and take action on any pertinent information you may discover along the way. Let's say, for example, that you had been taking 200 IUs of vitamin E daily because of a family history of heart disease. After discovering new research that suggests 400 daily IUs may be even more helpful, you discuss this information with your doctor, and then increase your daily dosage.

❏ Evaluate your goals. Determine if you have achieved what you set out to change.

Letting go of old destructive lifestyle habits while embracing new wellness patterns may not always be easy. However, many resources are available to help make your journey a pleasant one. Keep an open mind and learn as much as you can about health and wellness.

Lisa, one of my patients, had been diagnosed with lupus, a chronic and some-times fatal autoimmune disease. She was taking several medications, including prednisone, yet her symptoms of fatigue and joint pains did not subside. Her doctor told her that if she didn't stay on the medications, she would die from her condition. Lisa was scared half to death. One day, a friend of Lisa's suggested that she get an opinion from a nutritional doctor. Keeping an open mind, seventy-six-year-old Lisa made an appointment with my office. I prescribed supplements plus diet and lifestyle modifications, which eventually replaced her conventional meds. Today, Lisa is symptom-free.

When Lisa recommended this natural approach to several of her friends who were not getting any better with conventional treatments, they blatantly refused to get a second opinion. Since then, many of these friends have passed away without ever giving natural medicine a chance to improve their health or extend their lives. It is important to always keep an open mind to new ideas.

As your understanding of a healthy lifestyle grows, so will your awareness of the available options for achieving it. Libraries and bookstores, for example, provide many books, magazines, and audio and video tapes on health, fitness, nutri-

Sample Weekly Progress Chart

Goal	Activity	Action Steps	Feedback	Daily Points
Reach optimal weight.	Eat more carbs from heaven, eliminate carbs from hell.	Follow "7-Step Weight-Loss Plan" (page 191).	Loss of about 1 pound each week.	2
Increase water intake.	Drink 3 quarts per day.	Drink 1 quart (4 cups), 1 hour before meals.	Skin less dry; better bowel function; decreased appetite.	2
Eat more fruit and vegetables.	Adjust daily meals.	Include 2 fruits and 5 veggies each day.	Better bowel function.	2
Discover food addictions.	Maintain a diet diary.	Log foods eaten at each meal.	Elimination of symptoms caused by food allergens.	1
Exercise more.	Jog, walk, or swim 3 times per week.	Perform 30 minutes per activity.	Increase in energy.	2
Get a full night's sleep.	Get 7 to 8 hours of sleep each night.	Be in bed by 10 PM.	Increase in energy; a more positive attitude.	2
Feel more relaxed.	Laugh more.	Watch at least 2 comedy movies each week.	Increase in smiling; a more positive attitude.	1

tion, exercise, and psychology. Look inside your local newspaper for seminars or lectures on health and fitness, or wellness workshops that are available in your community. Seek out local or national organizations that promote health and wellness. Attending functions sponsored by groups such as the National Health Federation and the Vegetarian Society will put you in touch with others who are pursuing a wellness lifestyle like you.

Maintaining a week-long progress chart that includes and assesses your short- and long-term goals will help keep you on track and motivated. As you can see from the sample chart on page 161, specific goals are listed, along with steps for reaching them, and signs for assessing progress. Point values have also been assigned to each activity for evaluation. In this particular chart, an end-of-the-week total of sixty points is enough to gain a reward, which can be whatever you want it to be. You are in control. It's up to you to set up the point system, as well as the rewards. Just be sure to reward yourself with a treat that will reinforce your healthy lifestyle. Go see a funny movie. Visit a friend. Go to the art museum. Have dinner at a restaurant that serves gourmet healthy cuisine. (A blank "Weekly Progress Chart" for your convenience is presented on page 269.)

You're On Your Way

Establishing the first two steps of the "7 Steps to Living Well" will lay the groundwork for your journey to optimal health. It means your goals have been mapped out, along with a plan for tracking your progress. Hopefully, you have also found a good wellness coach to offer support and guidance. With the groundwork laid to form a strong foundation for your personal wellness plan, you can feel confident in moving forward to follow the next steps.

Chapter Ten

Eating Well

It goes without saying that eating a healthy diet is integral for achieving and maintaining wellness. This chapter presents Steps 3, 4, and 5 of the "7 Steps to Living Well." They offer solid dietary guidelines for good health. You'll discover which fruits and vegetables are at the top of the list for promoting wellness, learn how to best balance your intake of carbohydrates, protein, and fats, and find out about "power carbs"—concentrated whole foods that are packed with energizing vitamins, minerals, fiber, and phytochemicals.

Step 3. Eat a Rainbow

In order to reach wellness, you'll need to brighten up your plate and stimulate your taste buds with an assortment of vibrant-colored fruits, vegetables, grains, beans, and legumes. Eating dull-looking foods with little or no nutrition is one of the reasons many people are tired, overweight, and unfit. Foods that burst with color also happen to be rich in vitamins, minerals, antioxidants, phytochemicals, and fiber—the building blocks of wellness. The more colors, the merrier. Selecting carbohydrates from different color groups will provide flavor, eye appeal, and health-promoting nutrients. The following color guide will help you select the best produce at the supermarket, and encourage you to make healthy food choices whether you're at work, at home, or dining out.

Reds. Red is the color of love, fire, and passion. It is a hot choice when choosing your fruits and vegetables. When you include red or bright pink produce on your plate, such as tomatoes, red and pink grapefruit, watermelon, and guava, you are adding a potent antioxidant called lycopene. Scientists have discovered that this remarkable phytochemical significantly reduces the risk of certain cancers. After reviewing seventy-two medical studies, researchers at Harvard Medical School concluded that tomatoes reduce the risk of cancer of the prostate, stomach, pancreas, esophagus, breast, cervix, and lungs.

Red raspberries, sour cherries, and cranberries made the USDA's top twenty list of antioxidant foods. Scientists have also found that sour cherries have ten times stronger anti-inflammatory properties than aspirin—without the harmful side effects. Strawberries and raspberries contain *ellagic acid,* a phytochemical that hands a death sentence to cancer cells by neutralizing cancer-causing substances. Don't forget about red bell peppers and red grapes. Besides adding a colorful spark to salads and stir fries, they contain *anthocyanins,* powerful antioxidants and immune system stimulants.

Yellows and Oranges. Yellow is the color of hope and heartwarming sunshine. Fruits and vegetables that are yellow-orange in color, such as sweet potatoes, cantaloupes, carrots, mangos, and squash, not only warm the heart with their bright colors, they also promote good heart health. These carbs from heaven contain *carotenoids,* which help prevent LDL ("bad") cholesterol from sticking to artery walls. Carotenoids are responsible for the orange and yellow pigments.

Many citrus fruits that fall into this color category, including oranges, contain the phytochemical *hesperidin,* which helps prevent heart attacks and strokes by decreasing blood platelet stickiness. Oranges also increase HDL ("good") cholesterol, reduce LDL ("bad") cholesterol, and eliminate *homocysteine,* a harmful compound linked to heart disease. Last but not least, oranges contain phytochemicals that reduce the risk for liver, lung, and breast cancers.

Bright orange vegetables like carrots contain *beta-carotene*—a substance that the body converts into vitamin A. It also acts as an antioxidant and an immune system booster. Scientists have found that beta-carotene can decrease the risk of macular degeneration. And according to one study, eating just two carrots a day lowered cholesterol by up to 11 percent in the study subjects. Carb bashers want you to pass by the carrots at the dinner table. But now that you know better, you can take carrots to your health bank! Still not convinced? Scientists from the Harvard Nurses Study found that of the 80,000 women in the study, those who ate five carrots per week cut their risk for strokes by an astonishing 68 percent compared to the women who ate a scant one carrot per month—or none at all.

Blues and purples. Although blues and purples are the colors of tranquility and royalty, fruits bearing these colors are anything but peaceful when getting rid of harmful free radical compounds. In fact, blueberries and blackberries came in first and second respectively in the USDA's list of top fifty antioxidant foods. They eliminated more free radicals than any other fruits and vegetables on the list.

Then there are purple concord grapes. Scientists at the University of Wisconsin Medical School discovered that this majestic fruit safeguards the heart. First, these grapes prevent the narrowing and hardening of the arteries. Second, they reduce free radical damage caused by LDL cholesterol. Third, they help prevent heart attacks and strokes by reducing the stickiness of blood platelets. Red wine and grape juice that come from concord grapes also contain *resveratrol*—a remarkable protective compound that has shown potent antioxidant activity in the battle against free radicals. Scientists at the National Cancer Institute (NCI) are studying resveratrol's ability to inhibit cancer cells or even turn them back in normal, healthy cells.

Greens. The color green, which signifies prosperity, is the color of many varieties of produce that can pay big dividends at the health bank. Dark green vegetables are among the most aggressive disease fighters on the produce block. All of the cruciferous vegetables, such as broccoli, cauliflower, Brussels sprouts, cabbage, and kale, contain powerful cancer-preventive compounds.

Broccoli has a secret weapon called *indole-3-carbonol* (I3C), a phytochemical with potent anti-cancer properties. When broccoli gets in the ring with a cancer-causing substance, it packs a powerful knockout punch. Research scientists at Johns Hopkins Medical School found that broccoli inhibits the growth of breast cancer cells. Other scientific research has shown that it blocks the growth of several types of tumors. Recently, the National Cancer Institute announced that broccoli is Number 1 on its list of cancer-preventive compounds.

Earth Tones. Earth-tone colors are reminders of the beauty that is found in the simplicity of life. Beans and legumes come in a mosaic of subtle earthy colors, yet they pack as powerful a nutritional punch as vibrant-colored fruits and vegetables. Inside the color-coded coats of red kidney beans; white navy beans; brownish-pink pinto beans; yellow, orange, and green lentils; beige soybeans; and other beans of various colors, scientists have discovered antioxidants, flavanoids, and other cancer-protective compounds. Color is also important when choosing rice, bread, pasta, and beans. Unlike refined grain, such as white rice, bread, and pasta, which have been stripped of their color-rich fiber and nutrient-rich oils, whole grain cereals and breads have warm earthy tones, and contain vitamins, minerals, and phytochemicals that are heart healthy and cancer protective.

As you can see, there is much more to the color of carbohydrates than meets the eye. Fruits, vegetables, grains, and beans provide a kaleidoscope of colors; they are visually stimulating, and pleasing to our palates and well-being. Be sure to eat at least five to seven servings of fruits and vegetables per day (nine or ten would be even better). Select produce with the deepest, richest colors, since they provide the most vitamins, minerals, and phytochemicals. Eat generous portions of raw fresh fruits and vegetables—enjoy a colorful salad every day. To reduce your risk of diabetes, heart disease, and cancer, eat six to eleven servings of whole grains and beans daily. Take advantage of nature's bounty. Decorate and fill your plate with the rewarding colors of the rainbow. They will lead you to wellness.

Step 4. Balance Carbohydrates, Protein, and Fat

Each person has unique nutritional needs, yet there are some basic principles that apply to everyone. For example, everyone needs water. Similarly, everyone needs carbohydrates, proteins, and fats. A healthy eating strategy should include foods from each of these categories—restricting any one of them is a mistake. Keep in mind that man has relied on carbohydrates as a primary food source throughout history, yet obesity has rarely been a problem. People who blame obesity on carbohydrates are ignoring both history and science.

Time-proven evidence that plant-based diets sustain long-term health can be found in the extraordinary health of populations that eat the traditional diets of the Mediterranean, Asian, and Latin American regions. Carbohydrates have enabled countless numbers of people to maintain normal weight, while preventing long-term chronic disease. The following recommendations for carbohydrates, protein, and fats are based on the long history of dietary success enjoyed in these regions. They form the foundation of my American-MediterrAsian diet.

Carbohydrates

As I have shown in the earlier chapters, there are many reasons that the right carbohydrates are important for good health and well-being. The foundation of a healthy diet should include a large portion of carbohydrates from heaven (see the dietary guidelines in Chapter 13). Generous amounts of unrefined complex carbohydrates from fresh vegetables, fruits, whole grains, beans, and legumes should be included in the diet every day. Ideally, all carbohydrates from hell should be excluded, although an occasional intake is acceptable within a healthy eating strategy.

Above all, be certain to identify any carbohydrates or other foods to which you may be allergic. As explained in Chapter 6, the quickest way to accomplish this goal is through an ELISA allergy blood test. At the very least, follow an elimination/provocation diet (page 87).

Protein

Throughout the life cycle, protein—an essential nutrient—must be obtained from our food supply. Protein provides the building blocks for growth, development, and the repair of all body tissues. However, once the body's growth and development are completed, only small amounts of protein are needed for repair. (Athletes and pregnant women are exceptions.)

Most Americans eat far too much protein. How much protein do we actually need? The recommended daily allowance for protein for the average woman is 50 grams per day and 60 grams per day for the average man. This represents about a 30-percent margin of safety. The average American eats about 100 to 150 grams of protein per day. High-protein diets can easily include two to three times this amount.

Protein can be used as a source of fuel, but it is not efficient, nor is it clean. High-protein diets, especially those that derive protein from animal sources, create an extra workload for the body. Once protein is metabolized, nitrogen is released and toxic urea is left behind as a waste product. The urea must be processed and excreted by the kidneys. This extra work places a heavy burden on the kidneys.

Besides the extra strain high-protein diets place on the kidneys, the high saturated-fat content of animal protein makes them even more dangerous. An overwhelming amount of research has linked saturated fat to an increased risk in heart disease. In addition to saturated fat, once animal protein is metabolized, it leaves behind high levels of homocysteine. This toxic amino acid oxidizes cholesterol and promotes the formation of plaque inside the arteries. Arterial plaque buildup increases the risk for heart attacks and strokes. High-protein diets also increase the risk for gout, a form of arthritis. Protein can also raise insulin levels as much or more than carbohydrates. For example, beef can raise the level of insulin as much as 27 percent higher than whole wheat bread.

Fats

Just like carbohydrates, the composition of fats includes a backbone of carbon molecules coupled with hydrogen atoms. Different combinations of these two molecules determine the type of fat found in foods. Over the past two decades, dietary fats have been shunned by doctors and the general public. Anti-fat campaigns have been mounted by some of the nation's leading health organizations, including the American Heart Association. The USDA Food Guide Pyramid recommends that we cut back on all fat. But all fats are not created equal. Just as there are good carbs and bad carbs, there are also good fats and bad fats.

Fats are essential to good health and have several important jobs to perform. That is why certain fats are considered "essential." The body cannot manufacture them; they must be obtained through diet. Essential fats are vital to our health. For instance, the *cell membrane*, the outer layer of every cell, is made of essential fat. Essential fats allow nutrients to flow into the cell and waste matter to flow out efficiently. The *nerve sheath*, an outside protective covering around nerve cells and nerve fibers, is also made up of essential fat. In addition, sex hormones and body temperature are regulated by fats. If there is an insufficient amount of fat, these functions will be impaired Fats provide the raw materials for blood clotting and muscle contraction, and cause a feeling of fullness and satisfaction, which means you end up eating fewer calories.

There are four main categories of fat: saturated fat, trans fats (hydrogenated fat), polyunsaturated fat, and monounsaturated fat.

❒ **Saturated fats.** Found in high concentrations in animal foods, saturated fats are solid at room temperature. They raise LDL cholesterol levels, which can develop into fatty deposits called plaque. These plaque deposits can rupture, sending a piece(s) of plaque into the bloodstream, where it can block an artery and cause a heart attack or stroke. Research conclusively demonstrates that saturated fats increase the risk of heart disease, as well as certain types of cancer, such as those of the breast, prostate, and colon.

❒ **Trans fats.** Also known as hydrogenated fats, trans fats were originally liquid vegetable oils that were changed into a solid or a semi-solid state through a chemical process called *hydrogenation*. Trans fat products like Crisco vegetable shortening, margarine, and partially hydrogenated vegetable oils were created to sustain a longer shelf life than natural vegetable oils, which become rancid quickly. Researchers have found that trans fats are as bad, if not worse, for your heart than saturated fats. Hydrogenated fats are found in most processed foods, including crackers, cookies and most other baked goods; cereals; and potato chips and other snack products.

❒ **Polyunsaturated fats.** Considered essential fats because our body cannot manufacture them (they must be obtained through food), polyunsaturated fats are liquid at room temperature. (More detailed discussion on essential fats follows.) They are found in all raw nuts and seeds, fatty fish like salmon and tuna, and cold-pressed vegetable oils such as sunflower, corn, and soybean. These fats help to reduce the stickiness of blood platelets, which aids in the prevention of heart disease and stroke. In addition, omega-3 polyunsaturated fats help boost the immune system, decrease inflammation, promote eye and brain development and maintenance, reduce LDL cholesterol levels, and decrease blood pressure.

❐ **Monounsaturated fats.** Considered the heart healthiest, monounsaturated fats decrease LDL cholesterol and raise HDL cholesterol. Found in cold-pressed extra-virgin olive oil, canola oil, avocados, macadamia nuts, walnuts, almonds, and pecans, monounsaturated fats have several advantages over polyunsaturated fats. First, they are very heat stable—polyunsaturated vegetable oils are not. When exposed to high temperatures, polyunsaturated oils form harmful free radicals, which increase the risk of heart disease, cancer, and dozens of other illnesses and conditions. Both olive and canola oils can withstand high temperatures without forming harmful free radicals.

Monounsaturated fats do not compete with omega-3 fatty acids. This means monounsaturated fats do not disturb the body's normal balance of essential fats, which is further explained in the following discussion. Scientists have also discovered that monounsaturated fats decrease the stickiness of red blood cells, aiding in the prevention of heart attacks and strokes. In addition to offering all of these healthful advantages, monounsaturated fats make food taste better. And now for the best news! There is promising research that indicates monounsaturated fats may help encourage weight loss.

Olive oil is the primary fat used in the traditional Mediterranean diet, especially on the island of Crete, where it is reported that the "olive oil flows like wine." Yet, the people who live there have one of the lowest rates of cancer and heart disease in the world. No wonder there is so much excitement about their diet.

Fats That Heal

Certain fats have significant healing properties. *Essential fatty acids,* also known as EFAs, are fats that heal. Because the body cannot manufacture them, we must obtain EFAs from food. The two most important essential fats are omega-3 and omega-6. Omega-3 fats are found in pumpkin seeds, walnuts, dark green leafy vegetables, spirulina, chlorella, and cold-water fish, such as salmon, halibut, and trout. Omega-6 fats are found in cold-pressed corn, soy, sunflower, safflower, and sesame oils.

Essential fats are an integral part of every cell. They help form the outer membranes, which protect cells from attack by bacteria, viruses, and other foreign invaders. Cell membranes also allow nutrients to enter the cells and waste matter to be eliminated. To do this, they must be strong, yet flexible. Essential fats provide both of these properties. They are also necessary for the production of *prostaglandins,* local hormone-like substances that help regulate several body systems, including the circulatory and immune systems. As seen in the inset below, a deficiency of essential fatty acids can trigger many health problems. Scientist estimate that over fifty diseases may be linked to an EFA deficiency.

One of the keys to good health is the proper balance of essential fats. According to most health authorities, we should have a one-to-one, or at most, a two-to-one ratio of omega-6 to omega-3 fats. Diets with this ratio are among the healthiest populations in the world. Unfortunately, the average American follows a sixteen-to-one, and up to a twenty-to-one ratio. This amount of omega-6 fats in our diets is way out of proportion. To make matters worse, the omega-6 fats consumed by the average American are often toxic hydrogenated oils.

Although omega-3 fats play a vital role in health, they are severely deficient in the standard American diet. Omega-3 fatty acids produce local hormones that have anti-inflammatory properties. On the other hand, an excess of omega-6 fatty acids (which is common) produces local hormones that do not offer anti-inflammatory properties.

This excess encourages the development of inflammation and illness. Arthritis, inflammatory bowel disorders, and autoimmune disorders may be triggered by an excess of omega-6 fats, coupled with a deficiency of omega-3 fats. Researchers have also found that an excess of omega-6 fats may stimulate growth of cancer cells. The good news is that sufficient amounts of omega-3 fats can inhibit cancer

---

Results of Essential Fatty Acid Deficiency

The following is a partial list of the dozens of diseases and health conditions that scientists believe may be linked to a deficiency of essential fatty acids.

Angina	Eczema	Nervous system disorders
Allergies	Heart attack	
Arthritis	High blood pressure	Poor vision
Asthma	Infertility	Psoriasis
Cancer	Multiple sclerosis	Stroke

cells. Finally, scientists have observed that people with low levels of omega-3 fatty acids and an excess of omega-6 have an increased incidence of insulin resistance, a precursor of diabetes and heart disease.

Time for an Oil Change?

As you can see, balance between omega-6 and omega-3 fatty acids is essential for optimal health. The problem is that the average American eats a diet that is high in omega-6 fats and low in omega-3. Balancing the two fats can be a challenge for anyone, but there's good news. The age-defying American-MediterrAsian diet, presented in Chapter 13, makes it possible, practical, and enjoyable to obtain the proper essential-fat balance.

Trying to run your body on the wrong kind of fats is a big mistake. If you are not getting at least a two-to-one ratio of omega-6 to omega-3 fats, you are setting yourself up for chronic disease. Too much omega-6 fat and not enough omega-3 increases your risk of heart disease, cancer, arthritis, and a host of other degenerative illnesses. If you eat too much animal protein, not enough dark leafy greens or cold-water fish, and you do not eat flaxseeds, walnuts, or pumpkin seeds regularly, more than likely, your body is low on good oils—and it's time for a change.

Step 5. Take Advantage of Power Carbs

Whether you're a competitive athlete or simply a physically active person, power carbs can provide your body with a fuel that delivers peak performance. Power carbs are concentrated whole foods that are packed with vitamins, minerals, essential fatty acids, phytochemicals, and fiber, yet are surprisingly low in calories. Each power carb possesses unique healing properties. If you would like to have more energy, an enhanced immune system, improved digestion and elimination, decreased inflammation, and protection against heart disease and cancer—take advantage of power carbs. In addition to enhancing physical performance, they provide the brain with the perfect fuel for improved memory and concentration. They help maximize brain power and keep it mentally fit.

Carbohydrates are the primary source of fuel for the brain. The brain requires twice as much energy as any other body part, and power carbs provide it with a rich source of fuel and bioavailable nutrients. Unlike most foods, which take hours to digest and absorb, the nutrients within power carbs are quickly absorbed into the bloodstream and readily available in minutes.

These remarkable foods generate vibrant mental and physical energy, and help maintain a trim body that is more resistant to disease. Because they are nutrient-dense foods, power carbs provide optimal nutrition, which helps curb cravings for carbs and other foods. Doesn't it make good sense to provide your body with a concentrated form of fuel that can optimize mental and physical performance, while helping you lose weight at the same time?

So what are these power carbs? Available in health food stores, these products include bee pollen and royal jelly, essential sugars called glyconutrients, flaxseeds, Tahitian noni juice, wheat and barley grasses, and spirulina. Let's take a closer look at them now.

"Bee" Alive with Foods from the Hive

Bee pollen and royal jelly, products from the beehive, are two examples of nature's perfect foods. Bee pollen is 10-to 15-percent protein by weight, and contains all of the vitamins and minerals known to man. It also includes antioxidants, plant sterols, carotenoids and other phytochemicals, and several glyconutrients (see page 173). Interestingly, scientists have created bee pollen in the lab, but even though this man-made pollen contains the identical nutrients found in nature's version, bees die when fed it. Obviously, nature's bee pollen contains unidentified life-giving substances. Commonly used by Olympic athletes, bee pollen is a good choice for anyone who wants to increase stamina and fight fatigue, colon problems, depression, and cancer.

Scientists in Europe and Japan have done groundbreaking research on bee pollen and royal jelly. Dr. Peter Hemus, a cancer research scientist from the University of Vienna, found that female cancer patients treated with bee pollen had a "noticeable decrease in the side effects of radiation." He observed a marked decrease or a complete disappearance of nausea, loss of appetite, bladder irritation, and rectal swelling in the women who took bee pollen. Swedish research scientists, Drs. E. Ask-Upmark and G. Leander, observed that close to 80 percent of their patients with prostatitis and prostate cancer showed significant improvement after taking bee pollen for several months. Research conducted at several European universities found that males with a low sperm count showed a marked sperm increase and improved sexual performance after taking bee pollen for only one month.

Closer to home, Dr. William Robinson, a research scientist with the USDA, conducted animal studies that observed the effects of bee pollen on breast cancer in mice. In an article that appeared in *The Journal of the National Cancer Institute*, Dr.

Robinson reported that bee pollen slowed the growth of the breast tumors. He concluded, "[bee] pollen contains an anti-carcinogenic food." Dr. Leo Conway, a medical doctor from Denver, Colorado, has used bee pollen in his practice extensively. He found that patients who took three to five capsules of bee pollen per day "remained free from allergy symptoms."

World-class coaches have encouraged their athletes to take bee pollen for increased endurance and speed. When speaking of his former athletes, Tom McNab, former British Olympic team coach, novelist, and technical director of the Oscar-winning film *Chariots of Fire,* has said, "At least 90 percent of our athletes are taking bee pollen today. I think that bee pollen is the most effective, revitalizing food supplement available to athletes today, out of all the food supplements I have ever tested."

Royal jelly, another product from the beehive, is a thick, milky white, honey-like substance that worker bees provide exclusively for the queen bee. The worker bee lives about six weeks, while the queen bee lives about five years. The queen has extraordinary reproductive capabilities, laying about 2,500 eggs in a single day. The only difference between the workers and the queen is the food they eat.

Doctors in Europe and Japan use royal jelly as a medicine—an adjunct for fatigue, infertility, depression, and even cancer. Japanese researchers have discovered that royal jelly contains *royalisin,* a potent antibacterial protein. In one study, Japanese scientists induced sarcoma cancer into two groups of mice. One group was treated with royal jelly, the other was not. Compared to the untreated mice, the life span of the treated mice was extended by 20 percent, and tumor size was one half.

Although these products from the beehive contain a number of healthful benefits, they can cause allergic reactions in individuals who are sensitive to them. For this reason, bee pollen, royal jelly, and even honey should be used with some discretion.

Sugars That Heal

Many people are either not aware of or choose to ignore the fact that white table sugar, high-fructose corn syrup, and other refined sugars make kids climb walls, weaken the immune system, and contribute to heart disease for millions of Americans. It's hard to imagine, but the average American adult consumes about 130 pounds of refined white sugar per year, while children can eat more than twice that amount. Think about it. Most soft drinks have at least ten teaspoons of sugar in each can. There is an average of sixteen teaspoons of sugar in one piece of chocolate cake and thirty-two teaspoons in a banana split. It all adds up fast.

Numerous articles and books have brought a great deal of attention to the hazards of refined sugar, yet very few people are aware of the special group of eight essential sugars called *glyconutrients,* a name that means "sweet (glyco) nutrients." Don't worry; these sugars won't raise your blood sugar or insulin levels to make you fat. In fact, research indicates they will actually help you burn fat.

Scientists believe glyconutrients are one of the most important nutritional breakthroughs of the twentieth century. Only recently, there have been over 20,000 research papers written on them, with cover stories in prestigious journals like *Scientific American* and *Science Magazine,* and chapters in medical textbooks like *Harper's Biochemistry.* Scientists have discovered the remarkable ability of these extraordinary sugars to promote repair and regenerate injured or diseased cells by empowering the immune system.

Glyconutrients orchestrate communication between the body's cells, acting like a switchboard system that insures intelligent communication between cells, and allows every system to run in a smooth and orderly fashion. The body has a very complex communication network that connects every cell, organ, gland, and system, and arms them to defend against bacteria, viruses, and cancer cells.

Glyconutrients speak a universal language to all cells within the body. They help liver cells communicate with heart cells. They coordinate proper communication within the ranks of the immune system. They make certain the immune system destroys only foreign invaders like bacteria and viruses—without harming normal cells. They determine which minerals, fats, and other nutrients should enter the cells. And they help create digestive enzymes, regulate hormones, create mucous membranes to protect the digestive lining, and are involved in numerous other vital body functions.

Most physicians and dieticians think of sugar as nothing more than a source of fuel. However, new research is changing old thinking. Although your doctor may not tell you about glyconutrients for several years, you can take advantage of them right now. Currently, there are over forty pharmaceutical companies, spending billions of dollars every year trying to synthetically manufacturer these eight essential sugars. Ironically, they are many of the same corporations with sister companies that process foods and strip away vital nutrients, including glyconutrients, from our food supply. I find it quite interesting that these companies are working diligently to find a way to sell us "counterfeit" glyconutrients, while the genuine ones are already available in carbohydrates from heaven.

So, what are these eight glyconutrients and where are they found? They are glucose, xylose, mannose, galactose, fucose, N-acetylglucosamine, N-acetylgalactoseamine, and N-acetyleuraminic acid—long, complicated names that you don't need to remember. Just remember one thing. Glyconutrients are sugars that heal and bolster cell communication. They are found only in whole grains, seeds, mushrooms, the leaves of plants, and the roots, bark, and leaves of trees and shrubs. Some of the most concentrated sources of glyconutrients are brown rice, barley, oats, apples, oranges, grapefruits, onions, garlic, aloe vera juice, Tahitian noni juice, and mushrooms like Portabella, cordyceps, and shiitake—all carbohydrates from heaven.

Unfortunately, the average American rarely eats from this shopping list of carbohydrates. Scientists estimate that, at best, most people get only two of these eight essential sugars from the foods they eat. Although the body can manufacture the other six glyconutrients, doing so requires a significant amount of energy and great strain—a big expense. Although these essential sugars also come in supplement form, it is much wiser to obtain them from their natural sources—unrefined carbohydrates.

Flax: The Seed You Need

Flaxseeds are one of the oldest cultivated cereal grains. The first recorded use of flaxseeds as a food was in 3000 BC in ancient Babylon. Hippocrates, the Father of Modern Medicine, used flaxseeds for the relief of abdominal pain. Charlemagne, one of the most notable medieval kings, passed laws requiring the citizens of his kingdom to eat flaxseeds to assure they would receive the benefits of this remarkable food.

For centuries, flaxseeds have been used as medicine by many cultures throughout the world. They have served as laxatives, expectorants to soothe the linings of the throat and lungs, and external poultice to treat ulcers, abscesses, and inflammation. Most Americans, however, are unaware of this amazing sleeping giant of health foods. Typically, the small percentage of those who eat these seeds seek the benefits of its oil, and often overlook the advantages of the whole food.

So what is inside flaxseeds that makes them so special? An amount of 100 grams (5 tablespoons) of flaxseeds contains approximately 32 grams of essential fatty acids, 3 grams of saturated fat, 26 grams of protein, 4 grams of minerals, 9 grams of water, and an amazing 26 grams of fiber. Scientists have recently uncovered the healing properties hidden within these tiny seeds. They are a rich source of lignans, phytochemicals that, along with other phytochemicals found in flaxseeds, help strengthen the immune system to fight against foreign invaders like bacteria, viruses, and cancer cells. Lignans help block the absorption of estrogen, which aids in the prevention of estrogen-driven cancers like those of the breast, uterine, and prostate. Although lignans are found in other carbohydrates like wheat, barley, and rice, the content in flaxseeds is 200 to 800 times more concentrated than in any other plant known to man.

Flaxseeds have a high concentration of complete protein. In fact, the protein content is higher than that found in salmon. Flax also contains the mineral chromium, which helps regulate blood sugar and insulin levels. Chromium also helps decrease body fat and increase lean muscle mass.

Flaxseeds are the richest plant source of *alpha-linolenic acid*, the parent compound of omega-3 fatty acids. Although flaxseeds do not contain omega-3 fats, the body produces omega-3 fatty acids from alpha-linolenic acid. As mentioned earlier, an impressive amount of research demonstrates that omega-3 fatty acids boost the immune system, lower the risk of stroke and heart disease, improve brain function, and decrease inflammation.

Although it is wise to eat some flaxseeds every day, don't eat too much. They contain *cyanogenic glycosides,* a compound that contains a low level of toxicity. Small amounts of flaxseeds—4 to 6 tablespoons per day—contain a level of cyanogenic glycosides that is absolutely harmless. Flaxseed oil, however, does not contain cyanogenic glycosides.

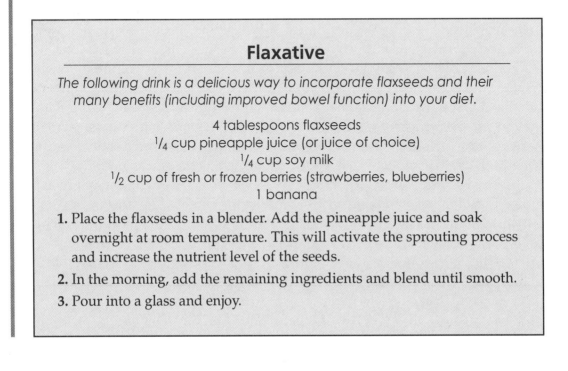

Flaxative

The following drink is a delicious way to incorporate flaxseeds and their many benefits (including improved bowel function) into your diet.

4 tablespoons flaxseeds
1/4 cup pineapple juice (or juice of choice)
1/4 cup soy milk
1/2 cup of fresh or frozen berries (strawberries, blueberries)
1 banana

1. Place the flaxseeds in a blender. Add the pineapple juice and soak overnight at room temperature. This will activate the sprouting process and increase the nutrient level of the seeds.

2. In the morning, add the remaining ingredients and blend until smooth.

3. Pour into a glass and enjoy.

Incorporating flaxseeds into your diet is simple. You can blend them into a fla-vorful drink (see page 176), or grind them up before adding to your favorite foods. Their nutty flavor is a delicious complement to cereals, salads, and a number of baked goods. You can also take flaxseed oil—two tablespoons per day (equivalent to four tablespoons of seeds) is recommended. The oil can be taken directly or added to salads.

Tahitian Noni Juice

"Nini nanna, nanna noni." This is not a Polynesian expression celebrating the ben-efits of the fascinating noni fruit. It is a little nonsense phrase that my nine-year-old daughter, Andrea, and I say to each other every day as I take the Tahitian noni juice from the refrigerator. Tahitian noni, or its botanical name *morinda citrifolia*, is a tropical fruit that grows in the unspoiled islands of French Polynesia. The juice of this fruit has helped the natives of Polynesian islands to live well for over 2,000 years. Today, millions of people are taking advantage of the miraculous healing properties of this amazing power carb from heaven.

Within the noni fruit, scientists have identified over 150 different phytochemi-cals, which is why it is able to help a wide range of health problems. For example, Tahitian noni juice contains plant *sterols,* phytochemicals that help slow down the absorption of "bad" cholesterol and elevate "good" cholesterol, boost the immune system, and decrease inflammation. Three of the most nutritionally important plant sterols are *beta-sistosterol, campesterol*, and *stigmasterol*. Tahitian noni juice con-tains all three.

Research studies demonstrate that the beta-sistosterol found in noni juice has anti-inflammatory and anti-cancer properties. It is not uncommon for people with arthritis to experience dramatic pain relief after drinking Tahitian noni juice. Men with enlarged prostates often find relief by taking the herb saw palmetto because it contains plant sterols. Noni juice contains much more than plant sterols, and it often works better than saw palmetto to relieve the symptoms of an enlarged prostate. Physicians who recommend noni juice for any chronic condition, includ-ing pain and inflammation, suggest it should be used for at least three months before evaluating its effects.

Whether you are young or old, noni juice helps promote healthy skin and hair because it contains essential fatty acids. These important nutrients, found in hair and skin cells, are often deficient in the standard American diet. Drinking noni juice not only helps maintain healthy skin and full-bodied, shiny hair, it also helps repair damaged hair and dry skin. From teenage acne to dull, lifeless hair, the healing properties of noni provide a welcome benefit at any age.

For over 2,000 years, native healers of the Polynesian islands have relied on noni juice as a remedy for pain, inflammation, fever, skin problems, bowel problems, and female disorders. They still prescribe regular consumption of the juice for the relief or elimination of common PMS symptoms, such as headaches, abdominal pain, bloating, and mood swings.

Although the native Polynesian healers have known for hundreds of years that noni juice helps many conditions, they didn't understand why. Today, scientists are uncovering some of these secrets. They have discovered that the most potent ingredient in noni juice is an extraordinary compound called *xeronine*. Dr. Ralph Heinicke, the research scientist who discovered xeronine, observed that it helps to regulate all chemical reactions inside the body by activating and recycling enzymes. Xeronine improves communication between enzymes, letting them know when to work and when to rest. It activates and potentiates hormones, and increases the absorption and uptake of all vitamins, minerals, and phytonutrients. Xeronine restores health by improving the body function's at the cellular level. New and promising research has also revealed that the xeronine contained in noni juice may be helpful in stopping addictions to alcohol, cigarettes, and drugs.

Dr. Heinicke has found that Tahitian noni is the richest source of xeronine, and a similar compound called proxeronine, known to man. Most fruits and vegetables contain small amounts of xeronine and proxeronine, with pineapple containing more than the others. But even pineapple is no match for the noni fruit. Three ounces of Tahitian noni juice contains the same amount of proxeronine found in one gallon of pineapple juice.

Dr. Neil Solomon, a researcher and former professor at Johns Hopkins Medical School, and the first Secretary of Health and Mental Hygiene for the state of Maryland, has done extensive research on Tahitian noni. In his book, *Tahitian Noni Juice: How Much, How Often, For What*, he documents his ongoing research. His study involves over 100 physicians and 20,000 patients who have benefited from Tahitian noni juice. Dr. Soloman found an overall average of 75 percent of patients benefited from this unique fruit. His specific percentages of improvement were documented as follows—asthma: 88 percent; arthritis: 80 percent; cancer: 69 percent; depression: 77 percent; fatigue: 90 percent; and fibromyalgia: 78 percent.

Tahitian noni juice is a virtual gold mine of disease-fighting phytochemicals. In addition to sterols and xeronine, it is a rich source of *scopoletin,* a natural anti-inflammatory, anti-histamine, anti-bacterial, and anti-fungal agent. Scopoletin also helps to regulate sleep, hunger, and body temperature. Noni also contains *damnacanthal* a powerful anti-cancer agent. Tahitian noni juice is considered an adaptogen similar to ginseng. Adaptogens help the body "adapt" to the unrelenting stress of modern life. There are only twelve known adaptogens—noni juice is considered the "premier" one.

Tahitian noni juice is a powerful immune system modulator. It not only boosts the immune system, it regulates it by intelligently reducing allergic responses, as well as autoimmune responses. Unlike prescription anti-inflammatory medications, such as Celebrex and Vioxx, noni juice is able to reduce pain without irritating the digestive tract, kidneys, or liver. In fact, noni juice repairs the digestive tract lining.

Wheat Grass and Barley Grass

Before a kernel of wheat or any cereal grass becomes a food from which we make flour, bread, or pasta, it passes through several stages of growth. Since 1930, scientists have known that during the early stages of the growth cycle, wheat, barley, and cereal grasses contain many times more nutrients than the mature grass. A study reported in *Journal of Agriculture Research* demonstrated that on the twenty-first day of growth (first joint phase), a field of barley grass contained 38.8 percent protein; on the forty-ninth day of growth (bloom stage), the protein content was 12.2 percent; and on the eighty-sixth day of growth (mature stage), the grass contained 3.8 percent protein. Young barley juice powder contains thirteen times more carotene than carrots, fifty-five times more vitamin C than apples, and five times more iron than spinach. After over 1,000 research studies, scientists concluded that during the first joint growth phase of wheat, barely, rye, and oat grasses, their nutrient content is essentially the same—extraordinary! The table on page 180 compares the nutritional content of wheat during the different stages of its life cycle.

Researchers in the United States and Japan have discovered that in addition to having a high concentration of protein, vitamins, minerals, and enzymes, young cereal grasses also contain phytochemicals, which have miraculous healing properties. Dr. Chiu Nan Laim, a research scientist from the University of Texas Medical Center, found that wheat grass juice inhibits the harmful effects of several cancer-causing chemicals. It also neutralizes the toxic effect of several dietary and environmental chemicals.

Nutrient Comparison of Wheat

The following table compares the nutritional content of wheat during the different stages of its life cycle. As you can see, "young" wheat grass is significantly more nutrient dense than whole wheat flour, which comes from "mature" grains.

Nutrients	Wheat Grass (100 grams dry weight)	Whole Wheat Flour (100 grams dry weight)
Protein	32.0 gms	13.0 gms
Fiber	37.0 gms	10.0 gms
Carbohydrates	37.0 gms	71.0 gms
Vitamin A	23,136.0 IUs	0.0 IUs
Chlorophyll	543.0 mgs	0.0 mgs
Iron	34.0 mgs	4.0 mgs
Calcium	277.0 mgs	41.0 mgs
Vitamin C	51.0 mgs	0.0 mgs
Folic Acid	100.0 mcgs	38.0 mcgs
Niacin	6.1 mgs	4.3 mgs
Riboflavin	2.03 mgs	0.12 mgs

In the table above, the following abbreviations are used: gm (gram), IU (international units), mcg (micrograms), and mg (milligrams).

In 1978, Dr. Y. Hagiwara, M.D., one of the world's leading authorities on the benefits of cereal grasses, demonstrated that barley grass is a powerful antidote for insecticides and food additives. At the 98th Annual Assembly of Pharmaceutical Society of Japan, Dr. Hagiwara presented his findings—barley grass was able to inactivate the agricultural insecticide Malathion. Barley grass extract reduced the concentration of Malathion from 100 parts per million (ppm) to 19 ppm in just two hours after incubation. The synthetic food preservative butylated hydroxytoluene (BHT), dropped from 400 ppm to 40 ppm after only five hours of incubation. Cereal grasses provide a serious protective shield against the hazards of chemical compounds in our environment.

Cereal grasses provide two powerful antioxidant enzymes called *superoxide dismutase* (SOD), and a fraction of SOD called *P4D1*. Both of these antioxidants slow down the mutation and deterioration of cells, making them valuable in the prevention and treatment of degenerative diseases and the reversal of the aging process. P4D1 has powerful anti-inflammatory properties, which scientists have discovered are more potent than the drug cortisone.

The carbohydrate configuration of cereal grasses has a large amount of *muco-polysaccharides* (MPs)—a substance that strengthens cell walls, lowers cholesterol, and reduces inflammation. Cereal grasses also have a high concentration of chlorophyll, the green pigment found in all plants and commonly referred to by scientists as the "blood of plants." There is good reason why green foods like cereal grasses are considered "blood builders." Some byproducts of digested chlorophyll may stimulate the production of blood cells in both animals and humans.

There is also some pretty impressive research that demonstrates chlorophyll has the ability to protect normal cells against the toxic effects of radiation and a wide range of chemicals. During the 1950s, the medical community routinely used chlorophyll as a medicine both internally and externally.

Spirulina: Nature's Appetite Suppressant

One of the most nutrient-dense plant foods on the planet, spirulina—a microscopic blue-green algae—is gaining widespread recent attention. It contains a powerhouse of nutrients and phytochemicals. Recently, there has been a flurry of research on this remarkable *functional food,* which is defined as any whole food that is able to improve the function of the body and prevent disease, while enhancing performance at the same time.

Spirulina is an ideal functional food with an unusually high level of quickly absorbable nutrients. It is rich in vitamins, chlorophyll, and phytonutrients; a concentrated source of protein (65 to 75 percent by weight); and a rich source of complex carbohydrates (up to 25 percent by weight). Spirulina is the richest plant source of vitamin B_{12}, and easily provides the recommended daily allowance for this vital nutrient. This is especially good news for vegetarians. It also contains significant levels of the essential fatty acid *gamma-linolenic acid* (GLA). GLA is a polyunsaturated fat that helps promote healthy skin and hair, decrease inflammation, and boost the immune system. Spirulina contains over fourteen minerals, including a rich supply of iron, and a full spectrum of natural carotene compounds, including beta-carotene.

Spirulina has a very high concentration of chlorophyll. It also contains complex carbohydrates, including fiber, and a rare carbohydrate (sugar) called *rhamnose*. This biologically active sugar has the ability to carry nutrients across the blood-brain barrier.

Drink Your Energy to Go!

These delicious power-carb drinks are a couple of my secret weapons against fatigue, food cravings, unwanted pounds, and illness. I have had one for breakfast just about every day for the past twenty-five years. I recommend them to all of my patients who are trying to get back on (or stay on) the road to good health. Each drink provides the remarkable benefits provided by both cereal grasses and spirulina. They are life-enhancing substitutes for coffee and caffeine-laden soft drinks. Very filling, they can also serve as meal replacements.

"Apple Pie" Go-Go Juice

12 ounces Knudsen's Spiced Apple Cider Juice* or Berry Juicy Juice
1 tablespoon barley grass powder
1 tablespoon spirulina powder

* You can also use plain apple juice mixed with $\frac{1}{8}$ teaspoon
cinnamon and a pinch of allspice.

1. Pour the juice into a mixing bowl. Add the barley grass and spirulina, and whisk until well mixed.

2. Although this drink tastes great, it looks as green as a lagoon, which you may find unappealing. Simply pour the drink into an opaque travel mug or sports bottle, and you will be good to go!

Blueberry Go-Go Smoothie

1 frozen banana
1 tablespoon spirulina
1 tablespoon barley grass powder
$\frac{1}{2}$ cup fresh or frozen blueberries
$\frac{1}{4}$ cup fresh or frozen blackberries
$\frac{1}{2}$ cup fresh-squeezed orange juice, or juice of choice
$\frac{1}{4}$ cup ice (optional)

1. Place all of the ingredients in blender and blend until smooth.

2. Drink slowly and enjoy every delicious bit of this power-carb drink, which looks and tastes great!

Researchers have also recently revealed spirulina's remarkable ability to lower cholesterol, strengthen the immune system, stop replication of viruses, and prevent and even reverse cancer cells. Because spirulina provides a rich source of nutrients, many physicians believe it acts like an appetite suppressant. Here's how. Hunger is registered in the brain. Since nutrient levels are significantly elevated after eating spirulina, the brain is subsequently tricked into thinking the body is full. And because spirulina also helps to maintain normal blood sugar and high levels of nutrients in the blood, it helps keep the appetite on an even plateau. The energy drinks found on the previous page, contain spirulina and barley grass, and can serve as meal replacements. They provide high levels of nutrients to curb your appetite, and subsequently reduce calorie intake to help you lose weight.

Multiple Vitamin . . . Inexpensive Health Insurance

Everyone knows that the average American diet is about as balanced as our national budget. Each year, the average person wolfs down 18 pounds of sweets and candy, 200 sticks of gum, 500 pounds of cakes, cookies, and biscuits made from refined flour and sugar, 63 dozen doughnuts, 20 gallons of ice cream, 5 pounds of potato chips, 150 pounds of refined sugar, 300 cans of soda pop, 30 pounds of French fries, and 3 to 5 fast-food burgers per week. It would take a good magician with a slight of hand or a crooked politician to balance numbers like these. Eric Schlosser, author of *Fast Food Nation*, claims Americans spend more money on junk food than on higher education, personal computers, or new cars.

"An apple a day" used to keep the doctor away—now it takes an apple and a multiple vitamin. A multiple vitamin is not a substitute for eating good food, but it can significantly supplement the shrinking levels of nutrients in our food supply. And they are shrinking, as seen in the chart on page 184. The question is no longer, "Do you need to take a multiple vitamin?" But rather, "Which multiple vitamin should you take?" RDA amounts are outdated. Today, you need ODAs—optimal daily amounts. It's impossible to get all of the nutrient ODAs in a one-a-day vitamin—unless it's the size of a horse pill. To get everything you need, it would take four to six pills per day. Look for a multiple vitamin and mineral that provides the following—calcium: 1,000 mgs; magnesium: 500 mgs; vitamin E: 400 IUs; chromium: 100 mcg; manganese: 5 mgs; zinc: 15 mgs; and B vitamins: 10 to 25 mgs. Be sure to choose a multiple vitamin with less than 10 mgs of iron unless a blood test indicates you have an iron deficiency.

Shrinking Nutrient Levels in Food Supply

The following chart shows the loss of certain nutrients in cabbage, broccoli, and onions between 1976 and 1997. The statistics are based on half-cup servings.

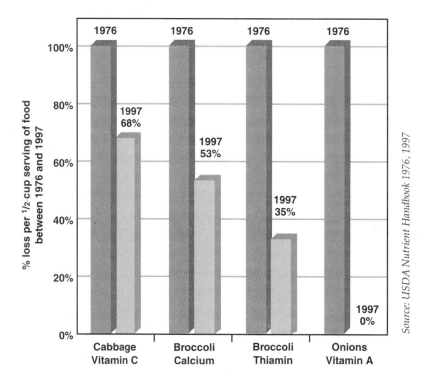

Source: USDA Nutrient Handbook 1976, 1997

You're Almost There

Steps 1 and 2, introduced in the last chapter, helped you set a solid foundation for climbing the "7 Steps to Living Well." This chapter showed how to continue the climb by detailing the important dietary guidelines found in Steps 3, 4, and 5. You're more than halfway to the top! The next chapter wraps it all up by presenting Steps 6 and 7. These final steps will help you discover the importance of exercise as well as a positive state of mind for a lifetime of wellness.

Chapter Eleven

Beyond Food

After eight to ten long hours on the job, most people are not enthused about "working out" at the gym. Does this sound like you? When you feel the urge to get up and exercise, do you lie back down on the couch until the urge disappears? If you are a couch potato, and you don't know how to get out of the rut, you're in for a pleasant surprise! Step 6 of the "7 Steps to Living Well" will show you how. Following this, the final Step 7 will explain the importance of laughter and a positive attitude in a life of wellness.

Step 6. Don't Work Out, Get Energized

Most people think of exercise as work, and this is where the problem begins. Why not change the way you look at exercise? Instead of calling it "working out," why not think of it as "a time to get energized?"

You are probably aware that exercise burns calories, sheds fat, and increases lean muscle mass. But did you also know that exercise generates energy, alleviates tension, and elevates mood all at the same time? It's true. Aerobic activity gets your blood pumping and oxygen moving throughout your entire body—and you get energized! Exercise gives you the mental and physical power to overcome stress, depression, fatigue, and illness. This type of strength makes you feel good about yourself—especially when you find yourself fitting into those "tight" clothes you haven't worn for the past few years. "But," you may be groaning, "Exercise is still *exercise*. Ugh." Although this may be true, there are ways in which you can overcome the negativity. The key is in choosing physical activities that are fun for you and that increase your heart rate at the same time. The tips and suggestions that follow should help you easily (and painlessly) incorporate exercise into your life.

Activate Your Daily Routines

Learn to incorporate physical activity into your daily routines. Try to be aware of ways in which you can add movement and energy to the things you do each day. Once you have this mindset and get into a rhythm, you will find yourself looking forward to finding new ways to include more movement in your life. But before you begin, you must first *turn off* your TV and *turn on* a commitment to living well. To get you started, here are some helpful suggestions that will get you off the couch and into motion:

❏ Instead of parking your car in the first row at work or as close to the mall entrance as possible, choose a spot in the last row. Then walk to your workspace or the store.

❏ Whenever possible, bypass elevators and take the stairs instead. Even sprint up a flight or two.

❏ Take your dog for a longer walk than usual.

❏ When you get home from work or school, don't plop yourself down in a chair. Turn on some music, grab your spouse, child, or a friend, and start dancing. And it doesn't matter if you don't know how to dance, just fake it! It's fun to listen to your favorite music while dancing (or trying to dance) a waltz, a line dance, the tango, a polka, the merengue, or the cha cha! Don't be so stiff—you're never too old to act like a kid.

❏ Whenever time and weather permit, take your bike to run local errands instead of the car.

These are just a few of the countless ways in which you can "energize" your daily routine. Once you get started, you'll be surprised at all of the new ideas you're going to come up with. Enjoy the challenge.

Make Exercise Fun!

Remember when you were a kid? When you ran and played all day without getting tired? How would you like to feel like a kid again, and have energy to spare? You will be glad to know that once you start eating power carbs every day and begin following the American-MediterrAsian diet (in Chapter 13), you'll be looking for new ways to spend the extra energy! And what better way to do so than through physical activities that make you feel like a kid again? Instead of "exercising," you'll be having fun—just like when you were young. You are never too old to play kids' games.

What follows are some classic games that take only minutes to play. You can enjoy some by yourself and others with one or more people. All can be played on the spur of the moment. They are great ways to "get energized" throughout the day. Try them in addition to your own favorites.

❏ **Frisbee.** This game is fun, inexpensive, and can be played just about anywhere—at a local park, the beach, or even in a small backyard. A frisbee is a round, flat, plastic object that looks like a dinner dish. Because you can throw a frisbee like a boomerang, you can play with it by yourself; however, it's a lot more fun to play with others. And no skill is required. Simply throw the frisbee to one another. You will quickly discover the fun of trying to catch the frisbee as it soars through the air. You'll find yourself running, stretching, and laughing—and best of all, you won't even realize you're getting energized. Playing frisbee will tone your upper body, thighs, and legs, and it's great for your cardiovascular system. Keep one in your car, backpack, or even your briefcase to have on hand whenever the opportunity to play arises.

❏ **Hula-Hoop.** Remember how much you laughed when you played with the Hula-Hoop as a child? This is another inexpensive and fun way to get energized and help shed those unwanted extra pounds around the waist. Some exercise experts claim that as few as ten minutes of Hula-Hooping each day for about a month, can help you shed up to two inches from your waistline. Just spin the hoop around your waist, hold your arms up in the air, and wiggle your hips in a circular motion. Try to see how long you can keep the Hula-Hoop in motion. Get ready to laugh and "hoop" it up!

❏ **Jump Rope.** This exercise may take you back to your days on the school playground. You can jump rope by yourself or with up to three people. The more the merrier. Start off slowly and work up to an aerobic pace. This is a great cardiovascular exercise that can be performed at any age. It's great for your heart, hips, thighs, and legs. For added fun, try jumping to some music.

❏ **Tag or Chase.** Tag is a universal game. It doesn't cost a thing to play, but pays great dividends. With moments of standing, sprinting, running, and darting, this game helps tone your thighs and legs, expand your lungs, and strengthen your heart. Get into the chase for the health of it!

❏ **Snake in the Grass.** This is my favorite family game, and a great way to get energized. We play it in our living room. First, we move our couch into the middle of the room. Next, someone volunteers to be the "snake," and then lies on the floor on his or her back. The other players then touch the snake's hands or feet with their feet. When the snake says the word "snake," the action begins. Everyone runs around the couch to get away from the snake—who is trying to tag them. As each person is tagged, they are out of that game. The game is over when all of the players have been tagged out. The first player to be tagged is the snake in the next game. The snake can chase the other players while standing on his feet, or, to make it more difficult, while on his hands and knees (wearing knee pads, of course). The game is fun and easy to play, and provides lots of excitement, laughter, and movement. You can set the pace of the chase to slow, medium, or fast.

Again, these are just a few examples of the many activities that make exercising fun. If you have children, get fit with them. In addition to being enjoyable, it offers a special opportunity for bonding. Busy work schedules and other time constraints often leave parents with little time for recreation, and children tend to spend too much time in front of a TV or computer monitor. Taking short breaks together is a perfect solution.

Step 7. Chuckle Every Day—To Keep the Doctor Away

If a chuckle a day keeps the doctor away, imagine what a bunch of belly laughs, several "goof-offs," and a couple of giggles can do for you. Chances are, you are not laughing enough. You have probably heard of illnesses that stem from vitamin deficiencies; however, you may be surprised to know that a lot of folks are suffering from a laughter deficiency. Everyone needs laughter—something I call "Vitamin HaHa."

A chuckle a day does keep the ills at bay. Mom talked about it, the Bible expresses it, and now science is actually proving it. Research is demonstrating that "a merry heart makes good medicine" (Proverbs 17:22). Scientists are just now catching up to this age-old Biblical truth. On the other hand, a laughter deficiency accelerates aging and increases the risk of serious health problems like cancer and heart attacks. In addition, it has been linked to hardening of the "attitudes," an increased risk of persistent anger and depression, difficulty in swallowing the humor of others, and a weakening of the "amuse" system.

The cure for laughter deficiency includes mega doses of Vitamin HaHa taken regularly. They will help buffer the stress of the hectic American lifestyle. It has been said that stress in our country is like a certain credit card. You can't leave home without it, and you can't stay home without it either. Stress has been implicated in many illnesses, including depression, insomnia, irritable bowel disorders, ulcers, and a weakened immune system. In fact, stress can be a killer. Most people experience too much unmanaged stress and too little laughter. This imbalance is one of the unrecognized causes of illness and hindrance to wellness. Laughter is a powerful stress buster.

Laughter is also a healthy response to life's hardships and inevitable challenges. Although it will not eliminate a problem, laughter will make coping with it more tolerable. It can soothe aggravation and turn a stressful situation into a comedy. Laughing in the face of adversity is a learned skill that anybody can acquire. Positive emotions are spirit lifters. Wouldn't it be interesting if doctors prescribed laughter instead of Prozac? Of course, this is not likely to happen; however, you can self-prescribe laughter on your own and take advantage of its benefits. Learn to loosen up and laugh more. Don't be afraid.

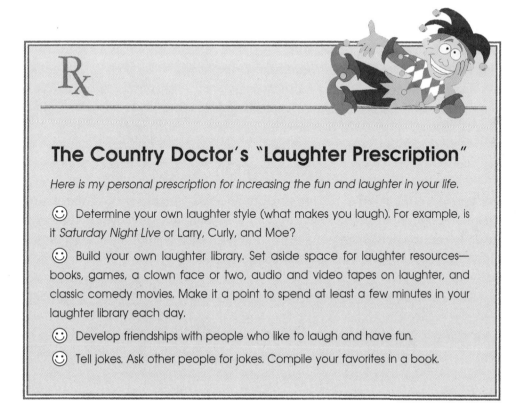

The Country Doctor's "Laughter Prescription"

Here is my personal prescription for increasing the fun and laughter in your life.

☺ Determine your own laughter style (what makes you laugh). For example, is it *Saturday Night Live* or Larry, Curly, and Moe?

☺ Build your own laughter library. Set aside space for laughter resources—books, games, a clown face or two, audio and video tapes on laughter, and classic comedy movies. Make it a point to spend at least a few minutes in your laughter library each day.

☺ Develop friendships with people who like to laugh and have fun.

☺ Tell jokes. Ask other people for jokes. Compile your favorites in a book.

Learning to laugh more will help you cope with stress, improve your health, and get you one step closer to wellness. The next time you are confronted with a stressful circumstance, try a shot of laughter. Don't get mad, get glad with this inexpensive, yet powerful medicine. Get in touch with "Doctor" W.C. Fields, "Doctors" Laurel and Hardy, and "Doctors" Larry, Curly, and Moe. These laughter specialists can provide mega-doses of laughter to brighten your day.

Make it a point to start each day by putting on a happy face. When you roll out of bed, be thankful that you're alive. Read a quick joke or a verse from an inspirational book. Compliment someone as soon as possible. Go out of your way to help others. Listen to happy songs. Be more like a child-taking time to play and laugh a lot! Tell jokes along the way. Make room for happy thoughts. Replace "stinkin' thinkin'" with uplifting thoughts. Here's a joke to get you started:

> A cat and three mice die and go to heaven. Saint Peter is standing at the pearly gates and asks the cat, "Tell me one special thing you'd like to have?" The cat says, "All my life I've wanted a cushy pillow. Could you give me a soft, cushy pillow?" Saint Peter says, "No problem. Come on in." Next, Saint Peter asks the mice, "If you could have one wish, what would it be?" All three say, "All of our lives, everyone has chased us. Could you give us each a pair of roller skates?" Saint Peter says, "Sure, we could do that. Come on in." A couple days later, Saint Peter is making his rounds and sees the cat sitting in the corner on his cushy pillow. He's got a toothpick in his mouth and is smiling broadly. Saint Peter says to the cat, "Hey, how do you like it up here?" The cat says, "Great! And I really like this pillow. But, I gotta' tell ya, I never expected the meals on wheels!"

Moving On

There you have them—the "7 Steps to Living Well." Incorporating these simple strategies—positive attitudes, healthy eating habits, and physical activities into your daily routine, will keep you on the road to wellness and help you maintain a healthy life.

Chapter Twelve

The 7-Step Knockout Weight-Loss Plan

L ife in the United States guarantees three things: death, taxes, and fad diets. Of the three, it sometimes seems as if fad diets get the most attention. Because of their round-the-clock battle of the bulge, Americans are continually searching for the perfect way to lose weight—and there is always a fad diet to offer false hope. There are many options. You can get into the calorie-restrictive Zone, blow bubbles in the bathtub with the Cabbage Soup diet, or experience "ketosis heaven" while eating bacon and pork rinds with the Atkins' Diet Revolution. But in the end, you will be disappointed—fad diets don't result in permanent weight loss.

Losing weight by restricting carbohydrates may work for a short period of time—but in the long run, it is the worst thing you can do. According to John Foreyr, Ph.D., a professor of medicine and psychology at Baylor College of Medicine in Houston, Texas, "When you get hungry, the first thing you think about are the foods you've denied yourself. You build them up in your mind until they become an emotional interference in your life, and then finally you binge." Most people who try low-carb diets end up in this predicament, but you can avoid this mistake by taking advantage of my American-MediterrAsian diet in Chapter 13. It is a diet based on thousands of years of success.

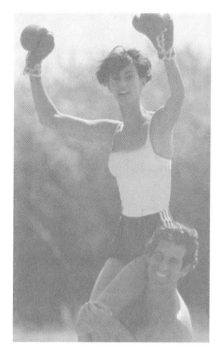

One guarantee comes with all fad dieting— when you go off the diet and resume eating the standard American diet (SAD), statistically, you will gain back all of the weight you lost and at least

5 percent more. Although we keep dieting, we continue to get fatter. In fact, we are on course to becoming the fattest nation in the history of civilization. During the 1980s, one out of every four people were overweight. Only a couple decades later, that statistic has become one out of every two!

It's hard to believe, but Americans are now reaching new levels of unhealthy eating as they wolf down French-fried Hostess Twinkees and double cheeseburgers that turn into double chins. When the binging is over, we end up spending over $33 billion dollars a year on worthless weight-loss schemes. Whether they are touting Fat Trappers or Exercise in a Bottle—a never-ending parade of infomercials

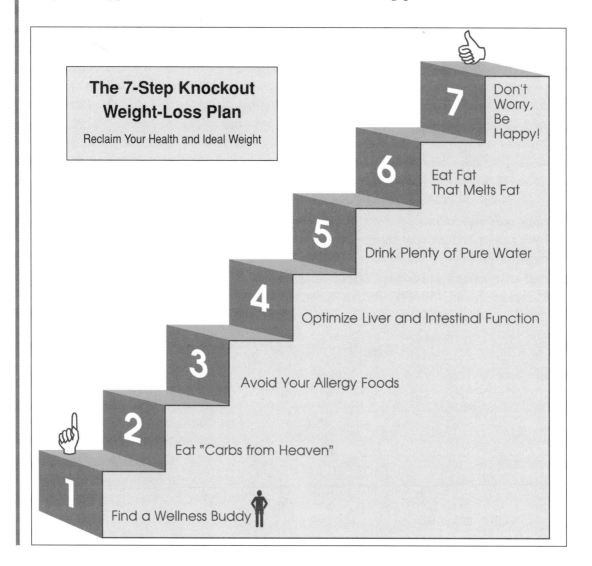

The 7-Step Knockout Weight-Loss Plan

Reclaim Your Health and Ideal Weight

7 Don't Worry, Be Happy!

6 Eat Fat That Melts Fat

5 Drink Plenty of Pure Water

4 Optimize Liver and Intestinal Function

3 Avoid Your Allergy Foods

2 Eat "Carbs from Heaven"

1 Find a Wellness Buddy

beckons us to try products that allow us to eat junk food while getting skinny at the same time. Others peddle pills or potions that guarantee bodies that look as if they've spent time in a gym. Desperate to try anything to lose those pounds, people blindly fall for these scams, never wanting to face the truth.

If you're tired of all of the weight-loss promises, gimmicks, and disappointments, I encourage you to stop dieting and change your lifestyle instead! It's your lifestyle that will determine your weight. If you eat double cheeseburgers regularly, you'll not only have a double chin, you'll probably have to have a double bypass as well. It's time for a reality check. Money can buy a lot of things, but it can't buy health. Good health, along with a fit and trim body must be earned.

Permanent weight loss begins with the right lifestyle choices. Long-term success comes from making healthy choices one day at a time. Permanent weight loss results from a different way of thinking. If you have tried a dozen different weight-loss programs and you're still overweight, it's time to admit to yourself that another diet *ain't gonna work.* Instead, you need to incorporate time-proven eating strategies that promote health, boost energy, and reduce the risk of degenerative disease. The right strategies will bolster your self-confidence and help you win the battle of the bulge. It's never too late! You can get started on your way to a lifetime of good health with a fit and trim body by putting the strategies found in the following "7-Step Knockout Weight-Loss Plan" into action. Enjoy the journey.

1 Find a Wellness Buddy

Old habits die hard! Changing your lifestyle can be a challenge—especially in the beginning. But when you have someone to share your wellness goals with, you are bound to be more motivated and ambitious in your quest. Sometimes will power is just not enough to help you change an old habit or initiate a healthy new one. It might take some extra support or a shot of encouragement from a "buddy" who cares about your well-being. Reaching out for help to achieve your goals is not a sign of weakness—it's actually a sign of strength and hope. A wellness buddy just might make the difference between the success or failure of meeting your fitness goals.

Since everyone is different and has unique personal goals, any successful wellness partnership must be flexible. Choose someone who has both of your best interests in mind and is willing to adapt to your needs. Wellness buddies may have different fitness levels and desired goals, yet they can still benefit from a partnership. From the start, it is important for each of you to be clear regarding what you expect to gain from the buddy system.

If you're trying to become fit and trim, the wellness buddy plan can help you stay on track to meet your personal goals. It may be just what you need if your goals don't match your ability to stay on track. There is power in numbers. Scheduling time to enjoy a swim, a bicycle ride, a walk in the park, a tennis game, or any other activity you may enjoy with family and friends is a good way to hold yourself accountable.

Being accountable to someone you love or don't want to disappoint is a key element to the success of any wellness strategy. According to the research of Jack Raglin, associate professor of kinesiology at the University of Indiana, couples that exercised separately had a 50-percent dropout rate after one year. On the other hand, couples that exercised together, regardless of whether they participated in the same activity or not, had a mere 10-percent dropout rate.

Your wellness buddy is someone who can show support by applauding your victories, laughing with you when you do something silly, prodding you out of your comfort zone, encouraging you to get back up no matter how many times you fall, holding you accountable to meet your goals come hell or high water, and celebrating your triumphs when you cross the finish line.

2   EAT "CARBS FROM HEAVEN"

I agree with low-carb diet doctors on one point—refined carbohydrates make you fat. As you have seen, carbohydrates from hell cause a rapid spike in blood sugar, raise insulin levels, and cause weight gain in a significant portion of the population. Refined grains are bad guys, but whole grains are good guys in the battle of the bulge. No matter how you cut it, a refined white flour bagel, stripped of most of its nutrients, is not the same as a whole grain bagel with all of its nutrients intact.

Yet most conventional doctors and dieticians consider all carbohydrates equal in the weight-loss equation. To them, a white bagel or a whole grain bagel is acceptable as long as it is eaten in moderation. This is because counting calories is the most important variable in weight loss according to the mainstream medical community. But let's face it, considering two-thirds of Americans are overweight, Dr. Atkins was right—the conventional weight-loss plan is not working.

If you want to shed those extra pounds and keep them off for good, one of the most important things you need to do is switch to carbohydrates from heaven. It's as easy as one, two, three:

1. Dump the junk carbs and eat generous portions of fiber-rich fresh fruits and vegetables, and unrefined grains, beans, and legumes instead. This does not mean you can never have any refined carbohydrates, just make an effort to minimize their intake.

2. Identify the carbohydrates to which you are allergic, and eliminate them for three short months. Then slowly rotate them back into your diet.

3. Eat until you are satisfied—not until you are full.

Carbohydrates from heaven pack a powerful punch when it comes to fighting fat. Scientists at University Hospital of London, Ontario, compared the weight and fiber intake of different individuals. They discovered that those who had a healthy weight ate 30 percent more fiber than the overweight individuals.

High-fiber foods can help you lose weight for a number of reasons. For one thing, you have to chew them longer, which slows down eating time. Fiber-rich foods have more bulk and fill you up faster with fewer calories. They also stabilize blood sugar levels, resulting in less insulin secretion, which translates into less weight. Furthermore, since we can't digest fiber, we can't absorb any calories from it either. The best form of fiber for weight loss comes from water-soluble fiber found in beans, legumes, oats, barley, fruits, and vegetables.

Food should be eaten for both health and pleasure. Switching to carbs from heaven does not mean you have to give up your favorite foods. Simply learn how to prepare your favorite foods with carbs from heaven. And yes, it is possible to turn good carbs into mouthwatering dishes! You won't feel deprived. In other words, you *can* have your cake and eat it too—as long as it is made with the right kind of carbs.

Instead of making your favorite pasta dish with white flour pasta noodles, use 100-percent whole wheat, brown rice, or whole corn pasta. One secret to great-tasting whole grain dishes, is to add generous amounts of extra-virgin olive oil. This eating strategy will satisfy your palate and enable you to peel off the fat without counting calories or fat grams. Be sure to eat 100-percent whole grain cereals that are sweetened with fruit juice instead of refined white sugar. Once you have lost a few pounds, go ahead and reward yourself with a guiltless dessert. Whole grain cookies, pies, and cakes are real foods that provide nutrients, fiber, and pleasure.

Be flexible, but try your best to eat carbohydrates from heaven most of the time. Eating healthy is determined by what goes in your mouth over time, not what you eat for one meal or for one day. And don't worry if you eat carbs from hell for a meal or two—it doesn't mean you've failed and there's no point in continuing to try. This kind of thinking is counterproductive and will sabotage your journey toward health and the body you want.

Be adventurous. Take your taste buds on a vacation by sampling foods from different cultures. There are countless recipes from around the world that include a wide variety of carbs from heaven and can add creativity, variety, and pleasure to your menu. Have you ever experienced the delectable flavors of a Greek meal, the robust flavors of Thai curry, or the savory goodness of a Mexican fajita? The culinary pleasures of Asia, India, and South America are tasteful adventures you will want to revisit time and time again.

Take a little time to plan your meals and snacks in advance. The extra effort will prevent you from resorting to junk food. Most important, be sure to create a meal plan that is satisfying to your palate. No one diet plan fits all people. Although I provide the American-MediterrAsian diet in Chapter 13, you can certainly create your own personalized diet based on the principles in this book.

3   AVOID YOUR ALLERGY FOODS

Do you have abnormal cravings for certain foods? Do you find yourself binging on your favorites? Do you commonly retain excess water or experience abdominal bloating? If you answered "yes" to any of these questions, you probably have hidden food allergies. Undiagnosed food allergies may be tacking on those unwanted pounds you have been carrying around for years.

Research scientists have discovered that if partially digested food finds its way through a weakened digestive lining and enters your bloodstream, food allergies and consequential weight gain can follow. Doctors have identified two main causes that trigger food allergies and weight gain—water retention and food addiction.

When partially digested food enters the bloodstream, it eventually finds its way into the tissues and organs, causing irritation and inflammation. The body then tries to reduce the inflammation by retaining water to dilute the concentration of toxic byproducts. During allergic reactions, *inflammatory prostaglandins* are also released. This class of prostaglandins can inhibit the body's metabolic rate and its ability to burn fat.

Unsuspected hidden food allergies can lead to food addiction, which, of course, will cause you to eat more and gain weight. In the October 27, 1979 issue of *The Lancet,* scientists observed that byproducts of allergic reactions act like *opioid-morphine* drugs, producing a temporary euphoric state, followed by a letdown, and then a craving for another food "fix." Over time, the allergic food is consumed so often, it can become physiologically and psychologically addicting. This is referred to as the food allergy/food addiction syndrome—and many people are trapped in it. Hidden food allergies eventually develop into uncontrollable food cravings, binge eating, and, consequently, weight gain. (See Chapter 6 for more on hidden food allergies.)

Recently, *The New England Journal of Medicine* reported that the opium-like compounds produced by food allergies increase appetite and decrease metabolism. As a result, the body's ability to burn calories is diminished, excess calories are stored as fat, and you gain more weight.

Carbohydrates and any other foods to which you may be allergic, could be the cause of your inability to lose weight. The old adage, "One man's food can be another man's poison," might be the answer to reducing your expanding waistline.

For nearly two decades, I have performed thousands of ELISA allergy blood tests. Through them, I have found that hidden food allergies are one of the major causes of weight gain. Although I don't consider myself a weight-loss doctor, I am confident that a beneficial side effect of eliminating allergic foods is weight loss. Patients routinely tell me that they had been unable to lose weight for years until we eliminated their hidden food allergies. And they lost the weight without counting calories or fat grams. Patients are always pleasantly surprised that they can actually eat more on their allergy-free diets than they've ever eaten before. In the inset on page 198, I share the story of one of my patients who shed forty-five pounds of fat as an indirect benefit of the treatment received in my office.

4 OPTIMIZE LIVER AND INTESTINAL FUNCTION

The liver is like a large manufacturing and processing plant. It is responsible for the production of digestive juices, blood proteins, and reserve fuel for the body. It also processes carbohydrates, fats, and proteins. The liver is the body's primary center for detoxification of environmental poisons and internal waste products; it is designed to remove impurities from the blood due to allergies, microorganisms, or chemicals.

The liver is one of the most overworked organs in the human body. Thousands of chemical reactions occur simultaneously within it every second. It manufactures 13,000 different chemicals, has over 2,000 enzyme systems, and is responsible for processing vitamins, minerals, and other essential nutrients.

The liver and the intestines have a symbiotic, cooperative relationship. Normally, the liver breaks down toxins and sends them to the intestines to be taken out of the body. If the bowel function is impaired by constipation or irritable bowel syndrome, waste matter is not eliminated properly, and toxins—chemicals, bacteria, and anti-

Shedding Twenty Pounds
of Phony Fat in One Month

Tim was very overweight and suffered with bloating, gas, and fatigue for as long as he could remember. When Tim was fifty-six, his cardiologist warned him that his elevated blood pressure, high cholesterol, and obesity put him at high risk for a heart attack. He told Tim that he had to lose weight. When Tim asked the doctor, "How do I do that?" the response was, "Just eat less food." For the next two years, Tim tried counting calories and eating much less food than he had in the past, but the weight did not come off.

When Tim came to our office, he hoped we could help alleviate his bloating, indigestion, and excessive gas. The possibility of losing weight wasn't even a consideration. I explained to Tim that his symptoms, including his weight problem, were probably linked to toxic reactions to foods. An ELISA blood test confirmed that Tim, indeed, had a number of food sensitivities. I put him on an allergy-free diet immediately. Within two weeks, Tim had lost all of his uncomfortable gastrointestinal symptoms, as well as twelve pounds of "phony fat" (my term for fat that results from hidden food allergies). During this time, he ate a wide range of foods, including potatoes and rice—two of the worst carbohydrates according to low-carb advocates. He also avoided the foods to which he was allergic, foods that he now calls "poison to my body." Tim later admitted, "I was very skeptical that eliminating foods I was allergic to could help my problems."

After one month, Tim had lost twenty pounds. Six months later, his weight loss totaled forty-five pounds! Just think. Participants in the recent Atkins' Diet research study at Duke University lost an average of twenty pounds in six months—whoopie! The study subjects had to severely restrict carbohydrates, and, according to Dr. Dean Ornish, noted expert on the diet alternative to heart bypass surgery, "They mortgaged their health to do it."

bodies from allergic reactions—are sent back to the liver through the blood. About two quarts of blood are filtered through the liver every minute. If the bowel becomes chronically constipated and toxic, eventually the liver will become overworked and unable to keep up with the toxic load. At this point, liver cells may become damaged and result in impaired liver function. The liver's filtration system can become congested and unable to efficiently remove toxins and fat. Liver congestion is similar to sinus congestion, although the waste matter in the liver is different from that of the sinuses. This can cause weight gain, fatigue, headaches, depression and other behavioral disorders, constipation, gallstones, recurrent illness, and even certain cancers.

How does liver congestion develop? When the liver is impaired and unable to process or eliminate waste matter efficiently, toxins enter into the bloodstream and set off alarms in the immune system. After repeated episodes of toxic overload, the immune system becomes overworked and unable to keep up with the ongoing assault. One consequence is weight gain, resulting from fluid retention as the body tries to dilute the toxic load. A more serious consequence of an overworked immune system is the possible onset of autoimmune diseases like arthritis, lupus, and multiple sclerosis.

Liver function can abort your weight-loss efforts in another, more direct way. Here's how. The liver produces *bile,* a fluid stored in the gall bladder. Whenever we eat any type of fat, bile is released from the gall bladder to emulsify the fat into tiny absorbable droplets. A congested liver, clogged bile ducts, or lack of nutrients can restrict the normal flow of bile, resulting in impaired fat absorption. Now, instead of breaking down fat, the liver stores it. You end up with a "fatty liver" plus roll of fat around your waistline—one sign of a congested liver.

The liver also breaks down carbohydrates into glucose, and stores excess sugar as glycogen. During exercise or when blood sugar levels suddenly drop, the liver converts glycogen into glucose for fuel to run the body. If there are not enough carbs in your diet, the liver will convert protein or fat into glucose for fuel. However, these sources of fuel are extremely inefficient and put extra strain on an already overworked liver—another reason that a low-carb, high-protein diet is not a good idea. Finally, a congested, overworked liver is unable to carry out normal blood sugar activities, which can lead to hypoglycemia (low blood sugar), sugar cravings, and weight gain.

As you can see, one of the most important yet overlooked solutions to permanent weight loss is a healthy, happy liver. Learning how to optimize liver function will go a long way to help you lose weight and keep it off. What follows are some practical tips on how to help maintain or restore normal function to both the liver and the intestinal tract. They will help you win the battle of the bulge.

❏ Eat Liberal Amounts of Carbs from Heaven

Fruits, vegetables, whole grains, beans and legumes, nuts, and seeds contain a magnificent combination of soluble and insoluble fiber. Fiber acts like an intestinal broom that sweeps out toxins processed by the liver and intestines. Water-soluble fiber also helps gather excess cholesterol and carry it from the body in the stool. Without a sufficient amount of fiber, cholesterol and bile are reabsorbed into the bloodstream and transported back to the liver, diminishing its fat-burning capacity. This is one of many reasons why I recommend beans and legumes so highly. The truth is, all of my patients are "full of beans."

❑ Avoid Refined Sugar and Artificial Sweeteners

Refined sugar and artificial sweeteners are a burden on the liver and intestines, increasing the risk of chronic disease. Refined sugar slows down *peristalsis* (muscular contractions) of the intestines, which can result in constipation and a toxic liver.

White table sugar (and other refined carbohydrates) raise blood sugar levels abruptly. Scientists at the USDA have found that refined carbs, like white bread and white pasta, spike blood sugar levels almost as quickly as white table sugar! Not only does this rapid influx of sugar burden your pancreas, it also makes your liver work overtime to convert the sugar into fats like triglycerides and cholesterol. Although the liver may make a gallant effort to process excess sugar, eventually it becomes overwhelmed, and fats begin to accumulate in it—and around your waist.

This reminds me of the classic *I Love Lucy* episode in which Lucille Ball is working on an assembly line in a chocolate factory. Because she is unable to box the chocolates fast enough, she starts stuffing them into her mouth, in her pockets, under her hat—everywhere but inside the boxes. Similarly, when it comes to extra fat in the liver, your body ends up stuffing it in places you don't want it.

❑ Avoid Harmful Chemicals

The accumulation of small amounts of food additives, pesticides, insecticides, preservatives, second-hand smoke, household cleaners, solvents, and heavy metals place extra stress on the liver and intestines. You can help protect these organs and lessen their workload by eating generous portions of fresh, unprocessed foods without harmful additives. Whenever possible, buy organically raised foods that are free from toxic herbicides and pesticides. Avoid public places that allow smoking. Use environmentally friendly cleaning concentrates, instead of commercial household cleaners that contain chemicals.

❑ Cut Back or Cut Out Caffeine

Have you ever tried skiing uphill? Do you ever bite your friends' fingernails? Have you ever chased your dog's tail? If so, you may be drinking too much coffee. Caffeine is a drug that must be processed and eliminated by the liver. Be kind to your liver. Try to reduce your intake of coffee or, better yet, eliminate it altogether.

Drink herbal tea or water instead. And be aware that coffee is not the only source of caffeine. Black tea, chocolate, soft drinks, a number of medications, and even some herbs, such as guarana, contain caffeine.

❏ Minimize or Eliminate the Use of Medications

After medications are broken down inside the body, their waste products accumulate in the liver. This means the repeated use of over-the-counter and prescription medications can cause potential liver damage. Cholesterol-lowering drugs are prime examples of these hazardous medications—patients who take them require routine blood tests to monitor liver function. As a culture, we have become dependent on over-the-counter and prescription medications. Comparatively, fewer people rely on safer, more conservative herbal and homeopathic remedies. Try substituting these safe, time-proven, natural remedies for conventional medications, especially over-the-counter varieties. Before stopping prescription medications, first consult with your physician.

❏ Minimize and Manage Stress

It has been said that stress is like a certain credit card: *"You can't leave home without it, and you can't stay home without it either."* Scientists have discovered that anger, fear, anxiety, resentment, jealousy, and other negative emotions trigger the release of harmful stress hormones such as cortisol. When stress hormones circulate in the bloodstream, they increase the production of fat and free radicals, placing an extra burden on the liver. Practice stress-management skills, like deep breathing, praying, meditating, and exercising. Try to do things that promote relaxation or encourage a lighthearted mood. Watching a good movie, strolling through the park, dancing the night away, or relaxing at the beach with a good book are just a few suggestions.

❏ Eat the Right Foods and Supplements

The liver and intestines have a remarkable capacity to repair and regenerate. Eating the right foods will encourage these actions and enhance their ability to function. Broccoli, cauliflower, Brussels sprouts, and kale, for example, contain *sulpheraphane,* a phytochemical that helps the liver neutralize toxins and eliminate them from the body. These foods are also high in fiber, which helps sweep toxins from the intestines.

The herb milk thistle is the most effective liver enhancer known to man. Turmeric is another. Milk thistle and turmeric are *lipotropic* herbs, which have the ability to slow down fat storage rate and increase the breakdown of fat in the liver.

Over 100 research papers have documented milk thistle's ability to repair, restore, and even produce liver cells. In large clinical trials involving thousands of patients, milk thistle has proved extremely effective in treating cirrhosis and fatty infiltration of the liver. Doctors in Europe routinely prescribe milk thistle for hepatitis, jaundice, alcoholic cirrhosis, inflammation of the liver bile ducts, and other liver disorders. Yet, this remarkable herb is safe enough for a pregnant woman to use without hesitation.

Garlic is another liver-friendly food. Like all beans, garlic provides sulphur-containing amino acids that assist the liver in removing toxic metals like lead, mercury, aluminum, and cadmium. Both beans and garlic aid in the production of bile.

Taking care of your liver and intestinal tract is critical for maintaining good health and optimal weight. Following the guidelines just presented will ensure that they are "healthy, happy campers" instead of your body's "tired, overworked employees."

5 DRINK PLENTY OF PURE WATER

You are bound to get really thirsty after what I'm about to tell you. Drinking an adequate amount of water can help you burn fat and shed unwanted pounds. Water is an essential factor of any successful weight-loss plan. To begin with, our bodies are 65 to 75 percent water. Insufficient water intake will cause the body to retain the supply of water it already has—and water retention can be responsible for as much as ten to fifteen pounds of excess weight.

Water is necessary to flush toxins from the kidneys and lymphatic system (a secondary circulation system that filters waste from the body). Insufficient water intake will impair the function of this vital body system. Many of the systems that keep our body thin require water. If any of them falter, we lose another fight in the battle of the bulge.

Without adequate water intake, metabolism slows down, energy levels plummet, toxins are trapped inside cells, and the body is robbed of oxygen and essential nutrients. According to scientists at the University of Utah, water is able to increase the body's metabolism by an amazing 3 percent. Their research also demonstrated that a 3-percent drop in metabolic rate from insufficient water intake translates into a pound of weight gain every six months.

Interesting new research indicates that once water enters the cell membrane, it produces energy that is not generated by food. Some scientists describe this energy as a kind of "hydroelectric power."

Replacing sugary, high-caloric drinks with calorie-free water is a guaranteed weight-loss practice you can take to the scales. The calories you drink are likely to end up as fat. One study found that individuals who ate an extra 450 calories in a day, adjusted their caloric intake by eating less at other meals, and did not gain weight. However, those study subjects who consumed an extra 450 calories from a cola drink, tended not to pay attention to those calories. As a result, they neglected to adjust their caloric intake at other meals and ended up gaining weight. The advantage of drinking water is that you can drink as much as you want and it won't turn into fat.

Don't fool yourself by reaching for a deceptively healthier sugar-free or diet soft drink, either. Artificial sugar-free sweeteners only compound the problem. They are metabolized into chemicals that lower blood sugar in the brain. Soon afterwards, hunger strikes. There is also evidence that these sweeteners may actually stimulate the appetite.

Although opinions differ on the amount of water we should drink, all health experts can agree that the average American is not drinking enough of it. In fact, the average American drinks a scant four-and-a-half cups of water per day. Most health experts suggest at least eight cups. The Mayo Clinic recommends that we drink half of our body weight in ounces of water per day. For example, if you weigh 200 pounds, you should be drinking 100 ounces of water daily. I encourage my patients to drink at least 96 ounces (three quarts) per day, no matter what they weigh. Whatever you decide is the right amount of water for you, be sure to meet your daily quota. It will help you reap many health benefits.

6   EAT FAT THAT MELTS FAT

Do I have your attention now? Is it possible that eating more fat will help you lose weight? Can you eat fat without having to worry about heart disease, cancer, and other diseases associated with aging? The answer to all of these questions is, "yes," but it all depends on the type of fat that you choose. Eating the right kind of fats and avoiding bad fats will help you to stay fit and trim, mentally sharp, and virtually free from the ravages of the "diseases of aging."

In addition to eating the wrong fats, restricting healthful fats is a guaranteed way to lose the battle of the bulge. Avoiding essential fats, which are good for you, is one of the reasons so many people binge on carbohydrates from hell and put on the extra pounds. Are you still skeptical? You're not alone. To most people, this sounds too good to be true, yet the research that proves it keeps mounting.

There are three types of fat that are necessary for maintaining a fit and trim body—omega-3, omega-6, and monounsaturated fats (MUFAs). Omega-3 and omega-6 fats are not produced in the body and must be obtained through the diet. Monounsaturated fats are not essential fats, yet they offer promising healthful benefits and aid in the fight against the battle of the bulge. As an added bonus, foods that contain monounsaturated fats taste great!

Oh My, Omega!

Omega-3 fatty acids are remarkable in that they not only help you shed fat, they dramatically reduce inflammation, prevent plaque buildup in blood vessels, decrease blood pressure, improve brain function, stabilize blood sugar, lower triglyceride levels, boost the immune system, and fight cancer. They increase the fluidity of cell walls to help transport nutrients and oxygen across the cell membrane and shuttle out waste matter.

Omega-3 oils increase metabolism and stimulate the production of enzymes that are required for burning fat and stimulating *thermogenesis*—a process that burns calories for heat. They decrease fat production and accelerate fat burning.

Remember, our bodies cannot manufacture omega-3 fats, so we need to acquire them from the foods we eat. Omega-3 fats are found in several carbohydrates from heaven, including soy beans, leafy green vegetables, flaxseeds, walnuts, spirulina, seaweed, and cold-water fish, such as wild salmon, tuna, halibut, and trout. Considering most Americans rarely eat these foods, is it any wonder that health experts estimate that up to 80 percent of our population is deficient in this essential fat?

Omega-6, another essential fat, is found in vegetable oils, like corn, sunflower, and safflower oils; however, consuming too much of this fat is not a good thing. Although the ratio of omega-6 fats to omega-3 should be two-to-one, the average American eats twenty times more omega-6 fat than omega-3—that's a twenty-to-one ratio! Way too much! This imbalance contributes to a number of health problems, including weight gain.

To further complicate matters, there are several factors that hinder the proper absorption of omega-3 and omega-6 fats, including hydrogenated oils, nutrient deficiencies, toxins, and viral infections. And although many people consume an excess of omega-6 fat, poor absorption can result in the deficiency of one of its important end products—gamma-linoleic acid (GLA). GLA is further broken down to form local hormones called prostaglandins. Prostaglandins made from GLA have the ability to reduce inflammation and burn fat calories.

This is precisely why alternative physicians typically recommend supplementing the diet with preformed GLA from omega-6 oils like evening primrose, black currant seed, and borage oil. Dr. Horribon, M.D., from the University of Montreal, observed that GLA-rich oils stimulate the thyroid gland and "rev up" the body's metabolism, which, in turn, burns fat. Plus, GLA mobilizes a special form of body fat known as *brown adipose tissue,* also called *brown fat.* Scientists have observed that brown fat burns fat calories—literally turning the body into a fat-burning factory.

The standard American diet is sadly deficient in omega-3 fats and the unrefined, unprocessed form of omega-6 fats. In order to reap the health benefits of these two essential fats, do the following:

❒ Eat unrefined carbohydrates from heaven, like leafy green vegetables, soy beans, flaxseeds, unrefined cold-pressed vegetable oils, and cold-water fish like salmon, halibut, tuna, cod, and trout. These foods are rich sources of unrefined omega-6 and omega-3 fats.

❒ Read food labels and eliminate all sources of hydrogenated oils, which contain harmful trans fats. Products such as margarine, salad dressings, commercial baked goods, potato and corn chips, and other snack foods fall into this category.

❒ Take a GLA supplement from borage, black currant, or evening primrose oil.

What Popeye Doesn't Want You to Know about Olive "Oyl"

Olive oil has gained a widespread healthful reputation, and although it will never replace Popeye's favorite food, this monounsaturated oil is a health food staple as well as a gourmet cook's delight. Recently, olive oil's reputation has been further enriched by some very promising research conducted at Harvard Medical School. In a study that involved over 100 subjects, half followed a high-fat Mediterranean-style diet, while the others followed a low-fat diet. After six months, those on the Mediterranean diet had lost almost 50-percent more weight than those in the other group—quite a significant amount. They also had almost a 50-percent lower dropout rate than those on the low-fat diet. In addition to weight loss, those in the high-fat group who had high blood pressure at the onset of the study, showed a reduction in blood pressure while on the diet.

What was most interesting about this Harvard Study is that both groups of participants ate plenty of fresh fruits, vegetables, and whole grains, with more than enough vitamins and minerals. However, the researchers observed that the participants on the high-fat diet ate more vegetables and grains, but surprisingly, 35 percent of their dietary fat came from monounsaturated fats. These heart-healthy fats came from foods like nuts, avocados, and olive oil—not from steak, sausage, and pork rinds.

A staple in the Mediterranean diet, olive oil is rich in antioxidants and can help the heart by lowering bad LDL cholesterol, maintaining and possibly elevating beneficial HDL cholesterol, and lowering triglycerides (fat circulating in the blood). A growing body of research shows that the right kinds of fats can help weight-conscious people lose extra pounds—and keep it off. This is great news, because in the long run, maintaining the proper weight will help lower heart disease and other degenerative illnesses.

In a nutshell, in order to lose weight and prevent degenerative illnesses like heart disease and cancer at the same time, eat fewer foods that are high in saturated fats. This means less meat and products made with hydrogenated fats, such as cookies, pie crusts, donuts, and other baked goods. Eat more foods with "healthy" fats, such as avocados, unprocessed nuts and seeds, olive oil, and cold-water fish. Following this type of high-fat diet is delicious and satisfying, and will promote weight loss that will last a lifetime.

7   DON'T WORRY, BE HAPPY!

It's no secret that too much stress can make you ill. But did you also know that stress can increase appetite and result in extra unwanted pounds? In the past, experts considered "comfort eating" merely a breakdown in will power. However, new scientific evidence indicates that when things go badly and you're tired, tense, or under pressure, reaching for those cookies, chocolates, potato chips, or other junk food can be triggered by a change in body chemistry that is brought on by stress.

According to Dr. Pamela Peeke, assistant clinical professor at the University of Maryland's School of Medicine, when we are faced with a stressful event or situation, the brain sends a message to the adrenal glands to release the hormones *adrenaline* and *cortisol*. These stress hormones trigger the release of glucose into the bloodstream. Glucose provides fuel for the muscles and increases the heart and respiratory rate. It also makes you alert and more focused. During certain situations, especially those in which you are faced with physical danger and must either fight it or escape from it, stress hormones can work to your advantage. For the average American, however, the release of these hormones is not usually prompted by physical danger, but rather by the increasing tensions of everyday life—your boss dumps an extra job on you, you're running late to catch a plane, your spouse forgets to complete an important task, you're stuck in traffic, or your teenager brings home a bad report card. These events also trigger the release of stress hormones into your bloodstream.

Any stress hormone elevation causes the release of glucose, which stimulates insulin production. Elevated levels of stress hormones signal your brain to fuel up the body as quickly as possible. This is a physiological green light that can cause an increase in appetite, especially for those carb-from-hell "comfort foods." During and after the mini-crisis, you can end up binging on the wrong carbs and tacking on extra pounds around the waistline.

What can you do to interrupt the consequences of stress? Instead of reaching for that sugar-coated comfort food, call up a friend, watch a funny movie, meditate, go for a swim, read an inspirational book, or play with your children. Do something pleasant that doesn't include consuming calories.

Take charge of the situation. Change your perception of the stressful event. Try thinking about someone else who is going through a more difficult challenge than the one you're facing. It won't improve the situation, but it will help reduce the amount of stress hormones that are being produced—and will minimize their appetite-stimulating effect.

Be happy. Do something physical—play a game of tag, jump rope, go dancing, or fly a kite. Physical exercise reduces the release of stress hormones and stimulates the production of the body's feel-good hormones, *endorphin* and *enkalphin*. Research demonstrates that exercise reduces stress, elevates mood, and burns calories (instead of adding them).

Finally, be sure to get enough rest. Sleep deprivation increases stress hormone levels. Not getting enough sleep also decreases the body's production of *leptin*, a hormone that triggers a feeling of fullness in the stomach. Jump-start your weight loss plan today by playing more and stressing less. Don't worry, be happy!
How about a couple stress-busting carb jokes? (You can see how determined I am to get you to smile and be happy.)

▨ *Trouble in the Ketchup Bottle* ▨

A little girl and her mother are in the kitchen preparing lunch. The little girl tries to get some ketchup out of the bottle to put on her sandwich, but it just won't come out. So the mother starts banging the bottle on the table to get the ketchup moving.

Just then, the phone rings. The little girl runs to the phone and picks it up. The pastor happens to be on the other end. "Hi honey, can I speak to your mom? "No," the little girl replies, "I'm sorry, my mom can't come to the phone right now because she's hitting the bottle!"

■ *Silly Wabbits Like Carrots* ■

A rabbit walks into a bar and says to the bartender, "Hey Elmer, what do you say? I'm really thirsty. Give me a tall glass of carrot juice." Elmer says, "You cwazy wabbit, we don't serve carrot juice here. This isn't a juice bar, you silly wabbit." So the next day, the rabbit walks back into the bar and says, "Hey Elmer, can't you see how thirsty I am? How about giving me just a small glass of carrot juice, will ya?" Now Elmer gets really upset and says, "You cwazy wabbit, I told you yesterday, we don't serve carrot juice, and if you ask me for it one more time I'm gonna nail your ears to the wall." So once again, the next day, the rabbit walks back into the bar and says, "Hey Elmer, got any nails?" Elmer says, "No, as a matter of fact we don't." So the rabbit says, "Heh, that's good news, Elmer. Give me a glass of carrot juice, will ya?"

Summing It Up

Remember, permanent weight loss begins by making the right lifestyle choices. Choosing to follow the "7-Step Knockout Weight-Loss Plan will help you win the battle of the bulge while promoting good health, boosting energy, and decreasing the risk of degenerative disease.

Part 4

The American-MediterrAsian Diet

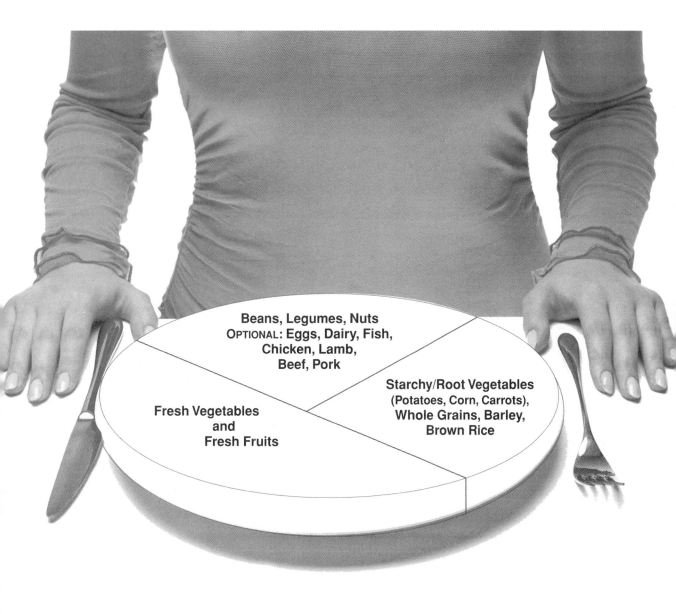

Beans, Legumes, Nuts
OPTIONAL: Eggs, Dairy, Fish,
Chicken, Lamb,
Beef, Pork

Starchy/Root Vegetables
(Potatoes, Corn, Carrots),
Whole Grains, Barley,
Brown Rice

Fresh Vegetables
and
Fresh Fruits

Chapter Thirteen

Prescription for a Healthy Lifestyle

Throughout this book I've encouraged you to ditch the carbs from hell, rely on carbs from heaven, and cut back on saturated fat. To enjoy the benefits of this eating strategy, I have blended three of the healthiest, most popular traditional diets from around the world—those of Latin America, the Mediterranean, and Asia (detailed in Chapter 8)—along with some healthy California cuisine, to create the American-MediterrAsian diet. This "intercultural experience" is not just another diet. It is a way of life that fosters a new appreciation for food, and a lifestyle that is centered around a table of enjoyment, appetizing meals, and good health.

Most people think eating healthy means being deprived of good taste. The American-MediterrAsian cuisine debunks this myth and proves that good health and great taste can be found on the same plate. Best of all, you won't have to put carbohydrate foods on a taboo list. Although the American-MediterrAsian diet is not a weight-loss plan—you *will* lose weight if you follow it. The diet's emphasis on fruits, vegetables, and whole grains, along with its sparing consumption of meat (eaten more as a condiment rather than a main event), will enable you to lose weight without even trying. The "7-Day American-MediterrAsian Menu Plan," provided in the next chapter, includes seafood, but not meat. After following the plan for one week, if you feel you would like to include meat in your diet, don't deprive yourself. Simply follow the guidelines for eating meat that are found in the American-MediterrAsian Diet and Lifestyle Pyramid on page 216.

Taking advantage of the time-proven benefits of the American-MediterrAsian diet and lifestyle will help you slow down the "aging" clock and experience a lifetime of wellness. But before presenting the details of this diet, it is important to first understand some of its inherent strengths. For starters, the American-MediterrAsian diet includes the right amount, balance, and types of carbohydrates, proteins, and fats. Also, many of its foods fight inflammation, which has been implicated in a number of chronic illnesses. Finally, the foods are delectable and satisfying—both nourishing and a pleasure to eat.

A Checklist to Stamp Out Inflammation

Until recently, inflammation had been associated only with conditions that end with the suffix "itis," like arthritis, colitis, bursitis, and diverticulitis. But in the early 1990s, scientists uncovered a connection between inflammation and most chronic illnesses and conditions, including obesity, allergies, Alzheimer's disease, heart disease, diabetes, and even cancer. The good news is that the prevention and cure for these illnesses may be closer than you think—like right in your own kitchen! That's right. You can actually squelch inflammation with the foods you put on your plate. Simply follow the dietary tips presented below. All are characteristic of the American-MediterrAsian diet.

❒ **Consume the right oils.** Monounsaturated extra-virgin olive oil, flaxseed oil, and the oil in most cold-water fish have potent anti-inflammatory properties.

❒ **Avoid carbs from hell.** Refined carbohydrates trigger inflammation.

❒ **Eliminate food allergies.** Foods to which you are sensitive/allergic cause toxic reactions and trigger inflammation.

❒ **Reduce or eliminate meat consumption.** The saturated fat found in meat increases the production of inflammatory prostaglandins.

❒ **Eat berries and cherries.** These fruits are powerful anti-inflammatory agents.

❒ **Spice up your life.** Culinary spices like rosemary, ginger, and turmeric, and green and herbal teas contain anti-inflammatory properties.

❒ **Lose weight.** Obesity increases inflammation.

"Good taste with a purpose." This phrase describes the anti-inflammatory aspect of the American-MediterrAsian diet. As an added bonus, by following this eating strategy, you will shed unwanted pounds and maintain a healthy weight. And because obesity increases the risk of inflammation, this is very good news.

Carbohydrate, Protein, and Fat Balance

The American-MediterrAsian diet provides the right amount and type of carbohydrates, protein, and fats. All three are necessary for maintaining a body and mind that are happy, healthy, and fit. The problem begins when we eat refined carbs, too much protein, and the wrong kind of fats. This diet provides a healthy balance of these three macro-nutrients in delicious and satisfying proportions.

❏ **Carbohydrates.** The American-MediterrAsian diet relies on healthy carbs from heaven, which will not make you fat. The suggested recipes, found in Chapter 14, incorporate an abundance of fresh fruits and vegetables, whole grains, beans, and legumes, to provide you with pleasure, energy, and a body that is fit and trim. The ingredients contain plenty of fiber and few calories. Consequently, it is possible that you can eat more food than you have in the past and still lose weight.

❏ **Protein.** Protein in the traditional diets of the Mediterranean, Asian, and Latin American regions is derived primarily from beans, grains, nuts, seeds, and fish; a small amount may come from chicken, beef, and/or pork. All three diets provide enough energy to build strength and endurance for sustaining an active lifestyle. Their emphasis on plant-based proteins while minimizing animal proteins prevents inflammation, which is implicated in weight gain and a number of illnesses.

❏ **Fat.** The fat content of the Mediterranean diet is higher than in the Latin American and Asian diets, yet all three provide protection against heart disease. Each derives an abundance of essential fats from vegetables, whole grains, nuts, and seeds, but the monounsaturated fats in the Mediterranean diet offer added benefits, like rich flavor and a satisfying feeling of fullness—ingredients for successful weight loss.

The American-MediterrAsian diet takes the guesswork out of eating "right." As you will see, following it is both easy and delicious!

Eat, Drink, and Be Merry

Mealtime should be a relaxing and enjoyable experience. Along with nourishment, food should provide pleasure and play a significant role in our social well-being. Pleasant conversation, music, and laughter should always accompany a good meal. To "eat, drink, and be merry" is part of the fabric of all cultural traditions, and actually aids in the proper digestion of a meal.

Every culture has unique tastes and traditions that are reflected in its foods. The cuisine of the American-MediterrAsian diet takes advantage of the healthy dietary traditions of three colorful global cultures. The menu plan found in Chapter 14 suggests a flavorful blend of these foods, and offers an opportunity to develop new food relationships. Especially when trying a new food for the first time, try to maintain an attitude that takes into account the interconnectedness between food, pleasure, and health. My goal in creating the American-MediterrAsian diet is to help you find pleasure in food and look forward to your next meal.

To add further enjoyment to meals, be creative. Arrange the food on your plate in an artistic manner. Be adventurous—discover smells, tastes, and pleasures you have never experienced before. The American-MediterrAsian diet helps you to expand your food repertoire. Remember, variety is the spice of life. Speaking of spice, learn to use spices and fresh herbs to add bursts of interesting flavor to your cooking. Eat at restaurants that serve natural food in a pleasant atmosphere. Plan a special meal with a friend at least once a week. Use festive tablecloths, candles, and fresh flowers. Play background music that fits the theme of the meal.

The American-MediterrAsian diet makes good health taste good. I realize that if you don't enjoy the food you eat, you probably won't eat it again (no matter how many health benefits it offers). You're going to love the American-MediterrAsian recipes. In addition to tasting good, they are void of artificial food coloring, chemical additives, refined sugar, refined carbohydrates, or excess saturated fat. Instead, you'll be eating meals that are prepared with disease-fighting ingredients that taste great. Good health needs to taste great—that's the American-MediterrAsian way.

Getting Started on the Path to Wellness

Alive with nutrient-rich foods, the American-MediterrAsian diet recommends dishes that are flavorful and fun to eat. The recipes are made with carbs from heaven, so you can eat your favorite foods, including some desserts, and still lose weight. As you will see, the road to good health does not have to be boring or cause you to feel deprived. It can be paved with taste-tempting fare that is both delicious and satisfying.

The material found in this section is designed to get you started on the dietary path to wellness. To begin, I have created the American-MediterrAsian Food Guide Pyramid and mapped out its dietary guidelines. I have also developed a flexible 7-day menu plan that includes a week's worth of healthy food suggestions, along with a recommended shopping list of ingredients to keep stocked in your pantry, refrigerator, and freezer. In Chapter 14, the traditional diets of Latin America, Asia, and the Mediterranean are represented in the recipe section, which includes easy-to-prepare dishes from these regions. (Some healthy California cuisine is also included.) I will show you how to cook with whole grain flours, beans, legumes, raw honey, unrefined sugar, soy milk, sheep and goat milk cheeses, fish, extra-virgin olive oil, and cold-pressed vegetable oils.

If you do not have time to prepare every meal outlined in the 7-day menu plan, don't worry. The inset beginning on page 221 lists the top fifty healthy fast foods—wholesome and delicious alternatives to foods made with carbs from hell. These good-for-you convenience foods are available in supermarkets and health food stores across the United States. Gardenburgers, okara patties (chicken substitute), and Boca Burgers (beef substitute), for example, are great-tasting alternatives to the all-American hamburger. Just pop them in the toaster or toaster oven and they're ready to eat in just minutes. Vegetable pot pies, pocket sandwiches, soups, frozen dinners, and desserts—all made with carbs from heaven—make staying on the American-MediterrAsian diet as easy as 1-2-3.

Time for a Change

The unexamined life is not worth living.

—Socrates

When we were children, other people in our lives decided what we should eat and drink, and when we should play. Unfortunately, even as adults, many people continue to base these decisions on the habits that were formed in their past. Most don't examine or question their current lifestyle, or reflect on their habits. What price does one pay for an "unexamined lifestyle" that is characterized by poor eating habits, high levels of stress, and little physical exercise? The answer is likely to be boredom, fatigue, illness, and possibly premature death.

One of the biggest reasons most people avoid self examination is because it requires change—fear of the unknown. However, a change in lifestyle could have a wonderful liberating effect. New experiences keep your mind and body fresh, enabling you to grow and become a better person in mind, body, and spirit. Everyone is searching for the fountain of youth. Yet the secret to youth has already been revealed. It comes from keeping an open mind, like a child. I'm surprised at how often people limit their experiences, especially when it comes to food choices. I encourage you to try new and different foods with an open mind and a willingness to let your taste buds make the decision.

Remember, the American-MediterrAsian lifestyle is not one that abandons pleasurable experiences at the dinner table, at work, or at play. Rather, it encourages replacing life's destructive habits with better, often more enjoyable ones. Take advantage of this lifestyle for at least one week. Try to incorporate all of the elements that are outlined in the pyramid (page 216). Consider it a vacation for your mind, body, and spirit. Approach the week with enthusiasm. You may be surprised to discover how good you can feel in such a short period. I'm confident that this experience will inspire you to make it a permanent lifestyle.

Energy-Packed American-MediterrAsian Diet

Based on the traditional diets and lifestyles of the world's healthiest cultures, the following American-MediterrAsian diet offers an eating strategy that is easy-to-follow, satisfying, and pleasing to the palate. Detailed guidelines are presented on page 217.

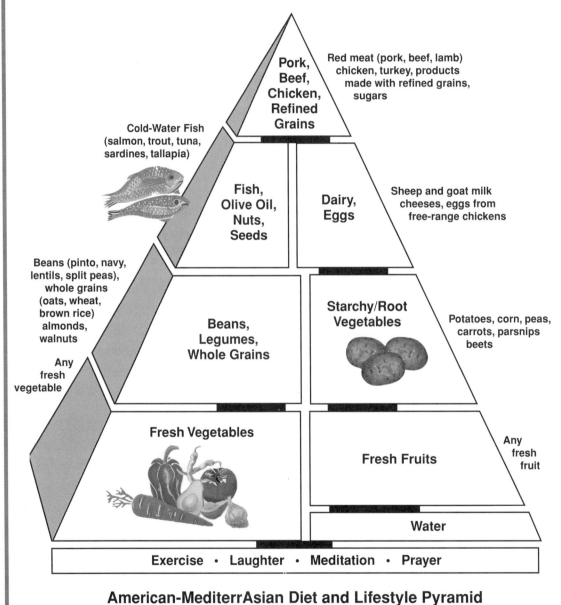

American-MediterrAsian Diet and Lifestyle Pyramid
Embracing the Joy of Health

American-MediterrAsian Dietary Guidelines

The elements that make up the American-MediterrAsian Diet and Lifestyle Pyramid on the facing page are further detailed below. As a general rule, always keep the following important guidelines in mind:

✔ Eat only when you are hungry.

✔ Eat to satisfaction, not to fullness.

CARBOHYDRATES

Eat three to six servings of whole grains every day. Choose from cooked whole grain cereal, coarse whole grain bread or muffins, and whole grain pasta.
One serving = 1 cup cooked whole grain cereal, 1 slice whole grain bread, 1 cup whole grain pasta.

VEGETABLES

Eat five to seven servings of fresh vegetables, either raw or steamed, every day. Vary your choices, but try to eat them mostly raw. If you cannot eat raw vegetables, try juicing them instead.
One serving = 1 cup raw vegetable or $^1/_2$ cup cooked.

FRUITS

Eat two to four servings of fresh fruit every day. For ideal health, eat a variety. Frozen fruit is acceptable, but it is not as nutritious as fresh.
One serving = 1 cup berries; 1 apple, orange, pear, banana, etc.; $^1/_2$ cup fruit juice.

PROTEIN

Required: Eat three to five servings of beans and legumes every day. Include choices such as pinto beans, kidney beans, chick peas, Great Northern beans, navy beans, white beans, black beans, soybeans, lentils, split peas, and black-eyed peas.
One serving = 1 cup cooked beans.
Eat $^1/_4$ to $^1/_2$ cup of nuts, such as almonds, walnuts, pecans, and filberts, every day.

Optional: Eat a maximum of 2 eggs, two times per week, and space them two to three days apart. Eat fish a maximum of three times per week; poultry, one time per week; and beef, lamb, or pork, one time per month.
One serving = A piece of fish or meat the size of a deck of cards.

Shopping List

Keeping your kitchen well-stocked with the right ingredients will make meal preparation easy and enjoyable. Although it isn't necessary to have all of the following items on hand, choose those that you and your family tend to like best. As you can see, there are plenty of options.

Stock Your Cupboards

Whole grains
Brown rice, oats, rye, barley, couscous, quinoa, corn.

Whole grain pasta
Bionature whole wheat pasta; Arrowhead Mills brown rice pasta, corn pasta.

Whole grain cereal
Barbara's, Grainfield, Peace Cereals, Mother's, Health Valley, and Arrowhead Mills brands.

Whole grain bread
White Wave, Ezekiel, Vermont, and Shilo Farms whole grain sandwich breads; Alvarado whole grain bagels and hamburger buns.

Dried beans/legumes
Pinto beans, kidney beans, navy beans, Great Northern beans, chick peas, lentils, split peas, white beans, black beans, soybeans, black-eyed peas. (Dried is preferred, but canned is acceptable in a pinch.)

Dried fruit (unsulphured, unsweetened)
Raisins, apricots, cherries, apples, prunes, pineapple, mango, dates, bananas, blueberries, figs, papaya.

Nuts
Raw almonds, pecans, macadamia nuts, walnuts, filberts, Brazil nuts, pine nuts, cashews, pistachios.

Raw seeds
Sunflower, pumpkin, sesame seeds.

Canned fish
Alaskan wild salmon, sardines in spring water, crabmeat in spring water, StarKist albacore tuna in water (contains no MSG or whey).

Canned tomatoes
Muir Glen fire-roasted tomatoes, tomato paste.

Bottled vegetables
Artichoke hearts, roasted red peppers, beets.

Prepared vegetable stock
Frontier Natural Products and Amy's brands.

Milk substitute
Silk soymilk, rice milk, almond milk.

Sparkling water
Pellegrino brand.

Herbal teas

Celestial Seasonings herbal teas; Good Earth Original caffeine-free teas.

Oils

Extra-virgin olive oil, cold (expeller) pressed canola or sesame oil.

Vinegars

Balsamic, red wine, white wine, apple cider.

Sweeteners

Unrefined cane sugar (Sucanat), raw honey, pure maple syrup, date sugar, unrefined molasses, stevia.

Soups (dry)

Fantastic Foods, Health Valley, and McDougal brands.

Condiments

Olives, pickled garlic, pickled ginger, stone-ground mustard, honey mustard, curry paste, barbeque sauce, ketchup, Bragg Liquid Aminos, Vegenaise eggless mayonnaise.

Herbs and spices, dried

Basil, oregano, parsley, sage, rosemary, thyme, cinnamon, ginger, garlic, curry, crushed red pepper, chipotle pepper, black pepper, sea salt.

Stock Your Refrigerator

Fresh fruits

All varieties.

Fresh vegetables

All varieties.

Soy yogurt

WholeSoy and Silk brands.

Soy luncheon meat substitutes

LightLife brand ham, bologna, turkey, salami, soy dogs, sausage, and hamburgers. Yves brand Canadian bacon, pepperoni, and ground "beef" varieties. These foods are advertised as soy meat substitutes.

Eggs

Organic or omega-3 enriched varieties.

Cheese

Sheep and goat's milk cheeses, such as Peccorino-Romano, Istara, Petit Basque, Kasseri, Manchego, French feta, Halloumi, Chevrie, goat-milk feta, Drunken Goat cheese, and Kashkaval. *Avoid cow's milk products, which commonly trigger allergic reactions.*

Fish

Alaskan wild salmon, trout, tallapia, orange roughy, sardines, herring, shrimp, scallops, oysters, ocean trout. *Fresh fish is highly perishable and should be eaten within twenty-four hours of its purchase.*

Stock Your Freezer

Frozen fruits
All varieties.

Frozen vegetables
All varieties.

Breakfast foods
Amy's brand Toaster Pops (apple, strawberry) and Breakfast Burritos. Lifestream brand waffles (seven-grain, buckwheat, mesa); Van's brand waffles (rice, seven-grain).

Pocket sandwiches and pot pies
Amy's brand pocket sandwich varieties, burritos, and pot pie varieties.

Entrées
Amy's and Celantano brands.

Fish
Alaskan salmon, trout, tallapia, orange roughy, sardines, herring, shrimp, scallops, oysters, ocean trout.

Vegetable burgers
Gardenburger, Boca, and Amy's brand veggie burger varieties.

Ice cream alternatives
Soy Delicious ice cream (Cherry Nirvana, Cookies Avalanche, Raspberry ala Mode, Butter Pecan) and ice cream sandwiches. Rice Dream ice cream bars and cookies.

Organic Eggs
Are They Really Better?

Are organic eggs really superior? See the difference for yourself. Break open an egg from a conventionally raised chicken onto a dinner plate. Now do the same with an organic egg. Observe the whites of both eggs. Notice how the the white of the organic egg forms a distinct raised layer, while the white of the conventional egg is thin and watery. This difference indicates the superiority of the protein structure of the organic egg, which also contains more nutrients.

Healthy Indulgences

What follows is a listing of fifty of the most popular but unhealthy convenience foods, along with a list of healthy substitutions. You will find that these great-tasting "heavenly" food alternatives are both wholesome and satisfying, and readily available in super-markets and health food stores across the United States.

Instead of Hellish Choices	Substitute Heavenly Alternatives
SNACK FOODS	
Potato chips	Kettle Foods and Guiltless Gourmet baked potato chips.
Corn chips	Skinny, Kettle Foods, and Guiltless Gourmet baked corn chips.
Pretzels	Barbara's and Shilo Farms whole wheat pretzels.
Rice cakes	Hain and Lundberg flavored brown rice cakes.
Crackers	Barbara's, Hain, Frookie, and Akmak whole grain crackers.
Pizza	Amy's nondairy pizza varieties; Kabuli whole wheat pizza shells (for making your own).
Finger foods (pizza bites, egg rolls, munchies, pierogies)	Health is Wealth nondairy baked dumplings, egg rolls, pizza and other "munchee" snack varieties.
French fries	Cascadian Farms baked fries.
Candy bars (chocolate)	Clif bars, Newmans Own candy bars; Tropical Source chocolate bars.
Milk chocolate chips	Sunspire Vegan Carob Chips or nondairy chocolate.
Hard candy	Glenn's peppermint swirls and lollipops; Tropical Source hard candies.
Yogurt (cow's milk)	WholeSoy and Silk soy yogurt varieties.

Instead of Hellish Choices	Substitute Heavenly Alternatives
DESSERTS	
Ice cream	Soy Delicious ice cream.
Ice cream cookies and sandwiches	Soy Delicious ice cream sandwiches; Rice Dream ice cream cookies.
Sorbet	Cascadian Farms sorbet varieties.
Popsicles	Cascadian Farms frozen sorbet bars.
Pudding	Imagine Foods and Mori-Nu puddings.
Applesauce	Eden and Santa Cruz organic applesauce.
MEATS/POULTRY	
Hot dog (all beef)	LiteLife soy Smart Dogs.
Hamburger	Gardenburger, Amy's, Boca, and LightLife burger varieties.
Chicken patty	LightLife soy chick'n cutlet; Natural Touch okara patty.
Fried chicken	LightLife soy chick'n burgers, cutlets, nuggets.
Italian sausage	LightLife Italian soy sausage.
Pork sausage	LightLife Gimme Lean soy sausage.
Meatballs	Nate's classic mushroom meatballs.
Ground beef	LightLife soy Gimme Lean or Ground Round; Yves Veggie Ground Round.
Bacon	LightLife soy bacon.
Canadian bacon	Yves soy Canadian bacon.
TV dinner	Amy's nondairy entrée varieties.
Beef burrito	Amy's nondairy burritos, tamale pie, enchiladas.
Paté, ham salad	Bonavita vegetarian paté varieties.
Luncheon meat	LightLife and Yves soy deli products.
Lunchables	Pete's Tofu brand "Tofu2Go."

Instead of Hellish Choices	Substitute Heavenly Alternatives
BREADS, PASTRIES, COOKIES	
Breakfast pastries, doughnuts	Amy's toaster pops; Van's and Lifestream whole grain waffles.
Pastries	Amy's, Barbara's, and Health Valley pies, tarts.
Cookies	Health Valley, Barbara's, and Midel whole grain cookies and granola bars.
Graham crackers	Midel and Morning Star whole grain graham crackers.
Breadsticks	Fattorie & Pandea whole wheat Italian breadsticks.
Bagels	Alvarado Bakery whole grain bagels.
DIPS, SAUCES, DRESSINGS, CONDIMENTS	
Dips and sauces	Fantastic Foods dip mixes.
Pickles	Cascadian Farm pickles.
Salad dressings	Amy's, Spectrum, and Newman's Own salad dressing varieties.
Salsa	Enrico's and Muir Glen salsa.
EGGS	
Egg salad	Mori-Nu Eggless Salad.
Scrambled eggs	Fantastic Foods Tofu Scrambler.
SOUPS	
Canned soup	Tabatchnick frozen soups; Fantastic Foods nondairy dry soups.
BEVERAGES	
Coffee with milk	Celestial Seasonings Roastaroma Herb Tea; Silk French Vanilla soy cream.
Milk (whole or 2%)	Silk soy milk; Rice Dream milk.
Milk shakes	Hansen; Naked smoothies.
Soda, sweetened fruit juice	Knudsen's fruit juice spritzers; Santa Cruz carbonated waters.

Time to Get Started

This chapter has spelled out the details of the American-MediterrAsian diet and lifestyle. Now that you have a basic understanding of this "recipe for a healthy life" (as well as a well-stocked kitchen to help you follow it), it's time to get started. The following chapter offers both a "7-Day Menu Plan" and a wealth of delicious, satisfying recipes that support the American-MediterrAsian diet. I'm betting you're going to be pleasantly surprised that eating "healthy" can taste so good!

Chapter Fourteen

Recipes for Good Health

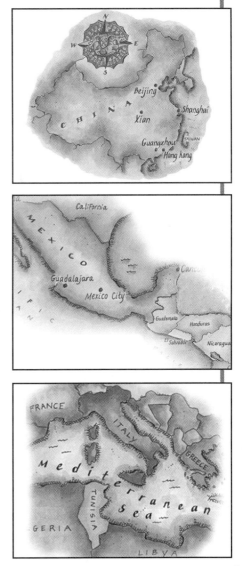

Based on the traditional cuisines of Asia, Latin America, the Mediterranean region, and a touch of California, the recipes presented in this chapter promote and support a healthy lifestyle—one in which carbs from heaven are enjoyed in abundance.

To help get you started on this eating strategy, the "7-Day American-MediterrAsian Menu Plan" on the next page suggests a week's worth of delightful food choices from the collection (or stockpile) of finger-lickin'-good "heavenly" recipes that follow.

This bounty of delectable international meals will keep you satisfied throughout the day. You can start out with a breakfast of piping hot Oat Pancakes or a Fruit & Granola Parfait. Try a Mexican Taco Salad for lunch, and enjoy taste-tempting Herbed Shrimp and Wild Rice for dinner. Looking for a snack? How about some Baked Wontons, Sesame Street Cookies, or a creamy Piña Colada Smoothie? Eating healthy never tasted so good!

In addition to promoting wellness, the American-MediterrAsian diet and lifestyle will help you lose those unwanted pounds—easily and, best of all, without feeling deprived.

7-Day American-MediterrAsian Menu Plan

The following menu plan includes fish, but no meat or poultry. After trying the plan for one week, you may decide that you would like to include these foods in your meals. If so, I encourage you to adhere to the dietary guidelines of the American-MediterrAsian Diet and Lifestyle Pyramid (page 217) for eating meat and/or poultry.

	Breakfast	Lunch	Dinner
DAY 1	Raspberry-Pear Breakfast Wrap (page 262), lemon-flavored herbal tea	Portabella Mushroom Sandwich (page 252), Baked French Fries (page 249), cut up raw tomatoes and bell peppers	Fiesta Chili "non" Carne (page 235), baked corn chips, green salad with South-of-the-Border Dressing (page 230), sparkling water with lemon
DAY 2	Oat Pancakes (page 229), fresh orange slices, Smoothie Ole'(page 237)	Bruschetta (page 241), Caesar Salad (page 245), spring water with lemon	Asian Poached Salmon (page 260), Roasted Rosemary Potatoes (page 248), Greek Salad (page 246)
DAY 3	Blueberry Breakfast Crisp (page 227), green tea	Fajita without the "Meata" (page 233), Quick Oil & Vinegar Salad (page 244)	Peasant's Secret Delight (page 249), sliced tomatoes and cucumbers
DAY 4	Frisco Bay Breakfast (page 228), Indian Fruit Salad (page 256), apple-cinnamon flavored herbal tea	Curried Tofu Sandwich (page 261), BBQ-flavored baked potato chips, lemon-lime spritzer	15-Minute Minestrone Soup (page 247), Caesar Salad (page 245), whole grain bread, water with lemon
DAY 5	Berry Delicious Smoothie (page 237), toasted whole wheat bagel with nonhydrogenated soy butter	Best Burrito Ever (page 232), cut-up raw carrots and cucumbers, baked corn chips	Skewered Singapore Tofu (page 260) over brown rice; cut-up raw carrots, bell peppers, and radishes
DAY 6	Fruit & Granola Parfait (page 240), coffee-flavored herbal tea* with French vanilla soy cream	West Coast Salmon Salad (page 231), baked potato	Mexican Lasagna (page 236), tossed salad with South-of-the-Border Dressing (page 230)
DAY 7	Nut-iterranean Smoothie (page 253), sliced strawberries	Thai Noodle Salad (page 256), sliced tomatoes and cucumbers, lemon-ginger flavored iced tea	Lentils with Caramelized Onions (page 251), Fattoush Salad with Whole Wheat Pitas (page 243)

Celestial Seasons brand Roastaroma is recommended.

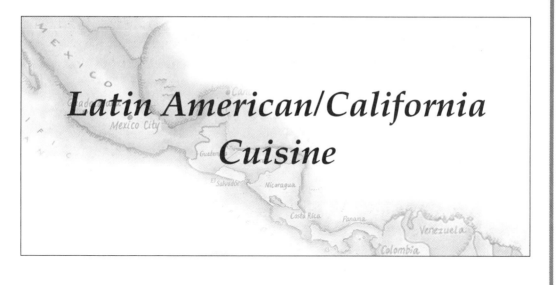

Latin American/California Cuisine

BREAKFAST FOODS

Blueberry Breakfast Crisp

3 cups cooked brown rice

3 cups fresh or frozen blueberries

1/3 cup Sucanat sugar

1/3 cup granola

1/4 cup whole wheat pastry flour

1/4 cup chopped walnuts

1 teaspoon cinnamon

3 teaspoons nonhydrogenated soy margarine or butter

8 ounces blueberry-flavored soy yogurt, such as Whole Soy brand

> Yield: 9 crisps
> (3-inch squares)

1. Preheat the oven to 375°F. Lightly coat a 9-x-9-inch glass baking dish with canola oil. Add the rice, blueberries, and half of the Sucanat. Stir well.

2. In a small bowl, mix together the granola, flour, walnuts, cinnamon, and the remaining Sucanat. Cut in the margarine until the mixture resembles a coarse meal.

3. Sprinkle the granola mixture over the blueberry-rice mixture. Bake for 20 minutes, or until the granola topping browns and the edges of the crisp are dry.

4. Serve warm, topped with some yogurt.

Frisco Bay Breakfast

This hearty skillet dish will help you start your day—in an ambitious way.

Yield: 4 to 6
servings

1 pound extra-firm tofu, frozen

2 medium potatoes, unpeeled and diced

2 tablespoons extra-virgin olive oil

1 clove garlic, minced

1/2 cup chopped onion

1/2 cup chopped green bell pepper

1/2 cup chopped mushrooms

3/4 teaspoon powdered thyme

1 teaspoon caraway seeds

2 tablespoons Bragg Liquid Aminos

1/4 teaspoon turmeric

1/4 – 1/2 teaspoon red pepper flakes, or to taste

Salsa or ketchup for garnish

1. Defrost the tofu, crumble, and set aside.

2. Boil the potatoes until cooked but slightly firm. Drain and set aside.

3. Place a large skillet over medium heat. Add 1 tablespoon of olive oil and the garlic, and sauté for 1 minute. Toss in the onion, sauté 2 minutes, then add the bell pepper and potatoes. Continue to sauté an additional 5 minutes. Add the mushrooms, thyme, and caraway seeds, and sauté 2 minutes more.

4. Heat the remaining olive oil and Bragg Liquid Aminos in a separate skillet over medium heat. Add the tofu, and sauté for 3 to 5 minutes. Add the turmeric and mix well.

5. Add the tofu mixture to the vegetables in the skillet. Sauté another 2 minutes, sprinkle with red pepper, top with salsa, and serve.

Oat Pancakes

These delicious pancakes are sure to bring about an appreciation of oats.

2 cups rolled oats

1 cup soy or rice milk

$1/2$ teaspoon cinnamon

$1/8$ teaspoon sea salt

2 tablespoons cold-pressed canola oil

> Yield: 6 pancakes
> (about 4 inches)

1. Grind the oats in an electric coffee grinder or blender until they are well ground, but not pulverized. (Small oat pieces add texture to the pancakes.)
2. Combine all of the ingredients except 1 tablespoon of oil in a medium-sized bowl. Let sit for one hour at room temperature.
3. Lightly oil a griddle and preheat over medium heat.
4. Pour about $1/3$ cup batter for each pancake. Cook about 1 minute, or until the tops are bubbly and the edges are dry. Flip the pancakes over and cook an additional minute, or until the bottoms are golden brown. Serve hot.

Breakfast Burrito

This mouthwatering Mexican-style breakfast wrap is hearty, delicious, and easy to make. As a variation, instead of mangoes and pears, you can use apple slices that have been sautéed in honey and cinnamon.

1 tablespoon extra-virgin olive oil

1 cup soy "sausage," such as LiteLife brand

4 whole wheat tortillas, such as La Tortilla Factory brand

$1\frac{1}{2}$ ripe mangoes, cut into strips

1 ripe pear, cut into strips

8 ounces strawberry-flavored soy yogurt, such as Whole Soy brand

Cinnamon to taste

> Yield:
> 4 burritos

1. Heat the oil in a skillet over medium heat. Crumble the sausage into the skillet, and sauté until brown.
2. Warm the tortillas in an unoiled skillet, and place on plates.
3. Place equal amounts of mango, pear, and sausage on the warm tortillas. Top each with yogurt and sprinkle with cinnamon. Fold the tortillas and serve.

Mexican Taco Salad

*This salad is a reminder of how similar the sunny flavors of
Latin America and the Mediterranean really are.*

Yield:
4 servings

8 cups chopped romaine lettuce

4 cups Fiesta Chili "non" Carne (page 235), or refried beans

1/2 cup tofu "sour cream," such as Tofutti brand

4 cups baked corn chips

1 cup salsa

1/2 cup grated Manchego cheese, or vegan soy cheese,
such as Vegan Rella brand

1/2 cup diced red bell pepper

1/2 cup diced yellow bell pepper

1/2 cup chopped black olives

1/2 cup chopped onions

South-of-the-Border Dressing (page 230)

1. On a large salad plate, layer the ingredients as follows: lettuce, chili, a few dollops of "sour cream," corn chips, salsa, cheese, bell peppers, olives, onions, and dressing.

2. Top with another dollop of "sour cream" and salsa, and serve.

South-of-the-Border Dressing

This Mexican vinaigrette will elevate the taste of any salad.

Yield: About
1/2 cup

1/4 cup extra-virgin olive oil

2 tablespoons red or white wine vinegar

1/2 teaspoon cumin powder

1/2 teaspoon chili powder

Juice of 1/2 lime

1/2 teaspoon lime zest

1/2 teaspoon Sucanat sugar

1. Place all of the ingredients in a blender, and blend until smooth.
2. Use immediately, or store in the refrigerator for up to two weeks.

West Coast Salmon Salad

The California influence on this great salad provides a welcome break from the usual "humdrum" dish. When time is a factor, you can use canned salmon instead of fresh.

12 ounces wild Alaskan salmon*
10 ounces spring mix lettuce or mixed baby greens
3 cups fresh strawberries
1/4 cup toasted pine nuts
Lemon wedges

Yield:
3 servings

* Do not choose farm-raised or Atlantic salmon.

DRESSING

3 tablespoons balsamic vinegar
3 tablespoons water
2 tablespoons extra-virgin olive oil
1 tablespoon Sucanat sugar

1. Place all of the dressing ingredients in a bowl and mix well. Set aside.
2. Cover the bottom of a large pan with water and add the salmon. Cover and steam for about 5 minutes. Carefully turn the salmon over and steam another 3 to 4 minutes, or until it is opaque and easily flakes with a fork. Transfer to a plate, and squeeze the lemon on top.
3. Place the lettuce, strawberries, and nuts in a large bowl, along with pieces of salmon and the dressing. Toss gently and serve.

Chipotle Mayonnaise

By increasing the amount of chipotle peppers, you can really turn up the heat of this flavorful mayonnaise.

Yield: About 1 cup

1 cup eggless mayonnaise, such as Vegenaise brand

1 teaspoon finely chopped chipotle pepper
with adobe sauce

1. Place all of the ingredients in a small bowl and mix until well blended.

2. Use immediately, or store in the refrigerator for up to two weeks.

MAIN DISHES

Best Burrito Ever

This burrito is an instant favorite with everyone who tries it.

Yield: 4 burritos

2 tablespoons extra-virgin olive oil

1 red or green bell pepper, sliced into strips

1 large onion, cut into rings

4 whole wheat tortillas, such as La Tortilla Factory brand

2 cups refried beans*

1 cup Chipotle Mayonnaise (above)

2 cups chopped romaine lettuce

Grated Manchego cheese or soy cheese, optional

* Use canned variety or easy-to-prepare box
of Fantastic Foods Refried Beans.

1. Heat the oil in a skillet over medium heat. Add the bell pepper, and sauté about 3 minutes. Add the onion, and continue to sauté another 3 minutes, or until soft. Remove from the heat and set aside.

2. Warm the tortillas in an unoiled skillet, then transfer to individual plates.

3. Place $1/2$ cup of refried beans and 2 tablespoons of mayonnaise on each tortilla. Add the sautéed onion-bell pepper mixture, lettuce, and cheese, if desired.

4. Roll up the tortillas and serve.

Fajita without the "Meata"

You won't ask, "Where's the beef" after biting into this hearty Mexican-style fajita. Our family usually enjoys them with a salad and side dish of rice. Instead of ground round, we sometimes use strips of soy "chicken."

2 tablespoons extra-virgin olive oil

12 ounces Mexican-flavored soy "ground round," such as LightLife or Yves brand

1 green pepper, cut into strips

1 cup sweet onions, cut into rings

4 whole wheat or corn tortillas, such as La Tortilla Factory brand

Salsa, to taste

Chipotle Mayonnaise (page 232), optional

Grated Manchego cheese, optional

Yield:
4 fajitas

MARINADE

$1/4$ cup teriyaki sauce

$1/4$ cup Bragg Liquid Aminos

3 tablespoons maple syrup

3 tablespoons fresh lime juice

2 tablespoons extra-virgin olive oil

$1/2$ teaspoon chili powder

$1/2$ teaspoon cumin

1. Mix all of the marinade ingredients in a bowl, and refrigerate for 2 hours.

2. Heat 1 tablespoon of the oil in a skillet over medium heat. Add the ground round, and sauté until browned. Remove from heat and set aside.

3. In a separate skillet, heat the remaining oil over medium heat. Add the green pepper and onions, baste with the marinade, and sauté for 3 to 5 minutes, or until tender. (You can also cook this on an outdoor grill.)

4. Stir the vegetables into the ground round, sauté another 2 to 3 minutes, and remove from the heat.

5. Warm the tortillas in an unoiled skillet, then transfer to individual plates.

6. Place $1/4$ cup of the ground round-vegetable mixture on each tortilla, and top with salsa. Add some mayonnaise and cheese, if desired. Fold the tortillas and serve.

Sloppy Joes

Yield: 2
Sloppy Joes

2 tablespoons extra-virgin olive oil

1 teaspoon minced garlic

1 cup chopped onion

3/4 cup chopped green pepper

8 ounces Mexican-flavored soy "ground round,"
such as LightLife or Yves brand

28-ounce can fire-roasted, chopped tomatoes, such as Muir Glen brand

3/4 cup smoked pineapple salsa*

2 whole grain hamburger buns

* If unavailable, use blend of 1/2 cup plain salsa, 1/4 cup crushed
pineapple, and liquid smoke (to taste).

1. Heat the oil in a medium-sized pot over medium heat. Add the garlic and sauté for 1 minute. Toss in the onion and green pepper, and sauté another 5 minutes. Add the ground round, and continue to sauté for 2 minutes. Stir in the tomatoes and salsa, and simmer the ingredients for about 2 minutes, or until heated through.

2. Spoon onto buns and serve.

California "Dagwood" Sandwich

Yield:
1 sandwich

2 slices crusted whole grain bread

1/2 ripe avocado

1 slice vine-ripe tomato

1 slice sweet onion

1/4 cup of alfalfa sprouts

1 teaspoon black olives

1 thin slice Manchego cheese

1 tablespoon Chipotle Mayonnaise (page 232),
or eggless mayonnaise, such as Vegenaise brand

1. On one slice of bread, layer the avocado, tomato, onion, sprouts, olives, and cheese.

2. Spread the mayonnaise on the remaining slice of bread. Place on top of the sandwich and serve.

Fiesta Chili "non" Carne

This versatile meal is a celebration of flavors. If you have any leftovers, use them as baked potato toppers!

2 tablespoons extra-virgin olive oil
1 teaspoon minced garlic
1 cup chopped onion
3/4 cup chopped green pepper
8 ounces Mexican-flavored soy "ground round," such as LightLife or Yves brand
28-ounce can fire-roasted, chopped tomatoes, such as Muir Glen brand
2 cups cooked kidney beans
2 cups cooked pinto beans
1 cup water
1 tablespoon unsweetened chocolate chips, such as Sunspire brand
1 tablespoon instant coffee substitute, such as Cafix or Roma brand
1 teaspoon dried oregano
1 teaspoon cumin
1/8 teaspoon cinnamon
1/8 teaspoon sea salt
Tomato juice, optional
3/4 cup smoked pineapple salsa*
1 tablespoon chili powder
1/4 – 1/2 teaspoon dried chipotle pepper, or to taste

Yield: 5 to 6 servings

* If unavailable, use blend of 1/2 cup plain salsa, 1/4 cup crushed pineapple, and liquid smoke (to taste).

1. Heat the oil in a medium-sized pot over medium heat. Add the garlic and sauté for 1 minute. Toss in the onion and green pepper, and sauté another 5 minutes.

2. Add all of the remaining ingredients except the salsa, chili powder, and chipotle pepper, and bring to a boil over medium-high heat. Reduce the heat to low, and simmer for 45 minutes, while stirring occasionally. If the mixture is too thick, add enough tomato juice to reach desired consistency.

3. Remove the pot from the stove, and stir in the salsa, chipotle pepper, and chili powder. Spoon into bowls and serve.

Mexican Lasagna

A dish like this is a reminder of how similar Mexican and Mediterranean cuisines really are. You can substitute vegetables like bell peppers or onions for the zucchini.

Yield:
4 servings

2 tablespoon extra-virgin olive oil

2 to 3 medium zucchini, cut lengthwise into $1/4$-inch strips

1 large sweet onion, cut into rings

12 whole corn tortillas, such as La Tortilla Factory brand

$1/2$ teaspoon chili powder

2 cups refried beans*

1 cup salsa

1 cup fresh or frozen corn, drained well

1 cup chopped black olives

1 cup grated Manchego cheese, or other
hard sheep or goat milk cheese

* Use canned variety or easy-to-prepare box of Fantastic Foods Refried Beans.

1. Preheat the oven to 350°F.

2. Heat the oil in a skillet over medium heat. Add the zucchini and onion, and sauté about 5 minutes, or until soft. Remove from the heat and set aside.

3. Arrange 4 tortillas on the bottom of a 9-inch square glass baking dish. Sprinkle with some of the chili powder. Spread half the refried beans over the tortillas, and layer half the zucchini-onion mixture on top. Add half the salsa, followed by half the corn, olives, and cheese.

4. Top with another 4 tortillas, and repeat the layers. Place the last 4 tortillas on top. If desired, top with more salsa and olives.

5. Bake about 25 minutes, or until the top is brown and the lasagna is hot and bubbly.

6. Cut into squares and serve.

Berry Delicious Smoothie

This refreshing smoothie is bursting with so much flavor, you'll forget you're drinking something healthy.

1 cup fresh or frozen blackberries

$1/2$ cup fresh or frozen raspberries

$1/4$ cup frozen apple juice concentrate

$1/2$ cup fresh-squeezed orange juice

1 frozen banana

$1/4$–$1/2$ cup ice

1 teaspoon raw honey

Yield: 2 servings
(12 ounces each)

1. Place all of the ingredients in a blender, and blend until smooth.

2. Pour into tall glasses and enjoy immediately.

Smoothie Ole'

This South-of-the-Border breakfast drink will make your taste buds say "Ole."

$1/2$ cup vanilla soy milk

$1/2$ cup coconut milk

1 frozen banana

1 teaspoon raw honey

$3/4$ teaspoon cinnamon

1 cup ice cubes

Yield: 1 serving
(12 ounces)

1. Place all of the ingredients in a blender, and blend until smooth.

2. Pour into a tall glass and enjoy immediately.

Piña Colada Smoothie

One sip of this delicious smoothie will transport you to a tropical island.

Yield: 2 servings (12 ounces each)

1 frozen banana

1 cup fresh or frozen pineapple chunks

$1/2$ cup vanilla soy milk

$1/2$ cup strawberry-flavored soy yogurt, such as Whole Soy brand

$1/4$ cup fresh-squeezed orange juice

$1/4$ cup unsweetened coconut milk

1 cup ice cubes

1. Place all of the ingredients in a blender, and blend until smooth.

2. Pour into tall glasses and enjoy immediately.

Lemon-Watermelon Cooler

A creamy and exotic tropical fruit drink—delicious and refreshing.

Yield: 1 serving (12 ounces)

$1\,1/2$ cups cubed watermelon

8 ounces lemon-flavored soy yogurt, such as Whole Soy brand

1 cup ice cubes

1 tablespoon fresh lemon juice

1. Place all of the ingredients in a blender, and blend until smooth.

2. Pour into a tall glass and enjoy immediately.

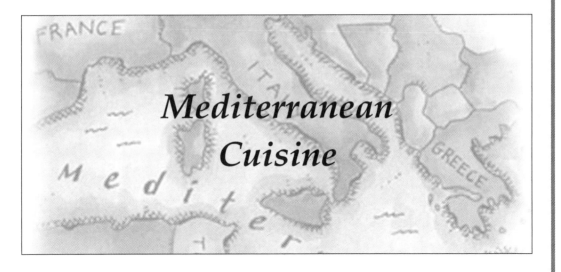

BREAKFAST FOODS

Couscous Breakfast Cereal

The mild taste of couscous in this breakfast cereal is brought to life with a touch of orange and cinnamon.

$^1/_2$ cup water

$^1/_2$ cup fresh-squeezed orange juice

$^1/_4$ cup soy or rice milk

1 teaspoon grated orange zest

1 tablespoon raw honey

1 tablespoon apple juice concentrate

$^1/_4$ teaspoon cinnamon

$^1/_2$ cup whole grain couscous

> Yield:
> 2 servings

1. Combine all of the ingredients except the couscous in a saucepan, and bring to a boil over high heat. Stir in the couscous, reduce the heat to low, and simmer covered for about 5 minutes.

2. Remove from the stove, fluff the couscous with a fork, and let sit a few minutes.

3. Serve plain or topped with some vanilla soy or rice milk, and a few berries.

Fruit & Granola Parfait

An extraordinary breakfast you can make the night before and enjoy first thing in the morning.

Yield:
1 parfait

$^2/_3$ cup fresh or frozen fruit, such as strawberries, raspberries, blueberries, or pineapple

$^1/_2$ cup granola

1 cup any flavor soy yogurt, such as Whole Soy brand

1. Place $^1/_3$ of the fruit in the bottom of parfait glass. Top with 3 to 4 tablespoons of yogurt, and 4 tablespoons of granola. Repeat the layers and top with yogurt.
2. Garnish with fruit and serve.

Herbed Scrambled Eggs

This classic Mediterranean dish will turn any breakfast into a festive occasion. Serve with a fresh fruit salad and some whole wheat toast.

Yield:
2 servings

4 large organic eggs

1 tablespoon extra-virgin olive oil

1 clove minced garlic

$^1/_4$ cup French feta cheese

1 cup fresh chopped spinach, optional

2 tablespoons minced fresh basil, optional

Black pepper to taste

1. Place the eggs in a small bowl, and beat with a fork or whisk. Set aside.
2. Heat the oil and garlic in a skillet over medium heat. Add the eggs, and cook about 1 minute, stirring occasionally.
3. When the eggs are nearly done, add the feta, basil, and spinach, if using. Continue to cook while stirring, until the eggs have reached the desired consistency.
4. Sprinkle with pepper and serve.

Bruschetta

This Italian favorite is more than an appetizer. Serve it with a salad for a light and refreshing meal. For a quick variation, do not cook the tomatoes or onions. Add the oil and 1/4 teaspoon balsamic vinegar.
Serve with or without the pesto.

1/2 teaspoon extra-virgin olive oil

1 clove garlic, crushed

1/2 sweet onion, chopped

1 large vine-ripe tomato, chopped

1/2 cup Pesto Sauce (page 242),
or Sun-Dried Tomato Pesto (page 243)

4 slices hard-crusted whole wheat bread

1/2 cup French feta cheese

1/2 cup pitted Kalamata olives

Black pepper

Yield:
4 servings

1. Preheat the broiler.
2. Heat the oil in a saucepan over medium heat, then add the garlic and sauté about 1 minute. Add the onion and continue to sauté 2 to 3 minutes. Toss in the tomatoes, and sauté another 1 to 2 minutes. Remove from the heat and set aside.
3. Toast the bread until lightly browned.
4. Spread 2 to 3 tablespoons pesto sauce on the bread. Top with 3 or 4 tablespoons of the tomato mixture, some feta, and olives.
5. Broil 5 to 10 minutes, sprinkle with black pepper, and serve immediately.

Pesto Sauce

This sauce is easy to make and bursting with flavor—a little goes a long way. Use it on pasta, pizza, or as a garnish for soups. Because this sauce is so versatile, I recommend doubling the recipe to always have some on hand.

Yield: About ½ cup

1 clove garlic, minced

½ cup chopped fresh basil, or 1½ tablespoons dried

5 tablespoons extra-virgin olive oil

⅓ cup pine nuts

1 tablespoon fresh lemon juice

1. Place all of the ingredients in a blender, and blend until smooth.
2. Use immediately, or store in the refrigerator up to two weeks.

Mediterranean Hummus Dip

This exceptionally delicious spread is a great dip for whole wheat crackers and pita bread, as well as raw vegetables. For added flavor, include one or more of the following ingredients to taste: dill, jalapeno peppers, black olives, and roasted red peppers.

Yield: About 2½ cups

16-ounce can chick peas, drained

⅓ cup sesame tahini

Juice of 1 large or 2 small fresh lemons

3 tablespoons extra-virgin olive oil

1 clove fresh garlic

⅛ teaspoon sea salt

1. Place all of the ingredients in a blender, and blend for about 1 minute or until smooth.
2. Use immediately, or cover and refrigerate up to 1 week.

Sun-Dried Tomato Pesto

This tangy pesto sauce is one of my family's favorite pasta toppings. It also adds a spark of flavor to sandwiches and soups.

1 cup sun-dried tomatoes

$1/4$ cup boiling water

5 cloves garlic

$1/3$ cup extra-virgin olive oil

$1/4$ teaspoon red pepper flakes, or to taste

1 tablespoon balsamic vinegar

1 tablespoon fresh basil, or $1/2$ tablespoon dried

$1/4$ teaspoon sea salt

Fresh black pepper to taste

Yield: About $3/4$ cup

1. To hydrate the tomatoes, place them in a small heatproof bowl and pour the boiling water on top. Let stand for 10 minutes.
2. Pour the tomatoes and soaking water into a blender along with the remaining ingredients. Blend only until chunky.
3. Use immediately, or store in the refrigerator up to two weeks.

SALADS AND DRESSINGS

Fattoush Salad with Whole Wheat Pitas

No Mediterranean menu plan would be complete without this exceptional mouth-watering salad.

2 large whole wheat pita breads

4 cups chopped romaine lettuce,

4 vine-ripe tomatoes, finely chopped

5 medium scallions, chopped

1 cucumber, finely chopped

1 green pepper, finely chopped

Yield: 5 to 6 servings

DRESSING

$1/2$ cup extra-virgin olive oil
Juice of 2 lemons
1 cup chopped parsley
1 clove garlic, minced
1 tablespoon dried peppermint
Sea salt to taste
Black pepper to taste
$1/2$–1 teaspoon dried sumac powder*

* Available in Middle Eastern food stores.

1. Cut the pita bread into small wedges and toast. Set aside.
2. Combine all of the dressing ingredients in a bowl and mix well.
3. Place the remaining ingredients in a salad bowl, add the dressing, and toss.
4. Add the pita wedges and toss lightly. Serve immediately while the pita is crisp.

Quick Oil & Vinegar Salad

This salad is a great starter for any meal.

Yield: 3 to 4 servings

2 cups chopped leaf lettuce
$1/4$ cup sliced cucumber
$1/4$ cup sliced tomato
$1/4$ cup diced green or red bell pepper
$1/4$ cup sliced onion

DRESSING

$1/2$ cup balsamic or apple cider vinegar
$1/4$ cup extra-virgin olive oil
1 tablespoon dried basil
$1/4$ teaspoon Sucanat sugar
$1/8$ teaspoon garlic powder

1. Combine all of the dressing ingredients in a bowl and mix well.
2. Place the remaining ingredients in a salad bowl. Add the dressing, toss, and serve.

Caesar Salad

A classic Italian salad with an optional splash of sun-dried tomatoes.

8 cups romaine lettuce, chopped

1 small sweet onion, sliced

$^1/_4$ cup sun-dried tomatoes, optional*

Caesar Salad Dressing (below)

1 cup whole wheat croutons

Yield:
4 servings

* If using sun-dried tomatoes, hydrate them in boiling water for 10 minutes.

1. Place the lettuce, onion, and sun-dried tomatoes (if using) in a salad bowl. Add the dressing and toss well.
2. Add the croutons and serve.

Caesar Salad Dressing

This classic salad dressing is meant for a bed of romaine lettuce, but it is also great on a baked potato.

$^1/_2$ cup grated Pecorino-Romano cheese

$^1/_4$ cup Dijon mustard

5 tablespoons plain soy yogurt, such as Whole Soy brand

5 tablespoons eggless mayonnaise, such as Vegenaise brand

2 tablespoons fresh lemon juice

$^1/_2$ tablespoon minced garlic

$^1/_2$ teaspoon Sucanat sugar

$^1/_2$ teaspoon Worcestershire sauce

Cayenne pepper to taste

Yield: About
$1^1/_2$ cups

1. Place all of the ingredients in a blender, and blend until smooth.
2. Use immediately, or refrigerate for up to 1 week.

Greek Salad

This colorful version of a Greek salad adds a slight twist to a traditional Mediterranean favorite. Try it with Lentils with Caramelized Onions (page 251) and Roasted Rosemary Potatoes (page 248).

Yield:
5 servings

5 cups chopped romaine lettuce

1 vine-ripe tomato, diced

1/4 sweet onion, sliced

1/2 cup cooked sliced beets

1/2 cup crumbled French feta cheese

1/3 cup cooked chick peas

DRESSING

1/4 cup extra-virgin olive oil

1/4 cup balsamic vinegar

1/3 cup sliced Kalamata olives and 1/4 cup juice

1 teaspoon dried oregano

1/4 teaspoon black pepper, or to taste

1. Combine all of the dressing ingredients in a bowl and mix well.
2. Place the remaining ingredients in a salad bowl, add the dressing, and toss well. Serve immediately.

15-Minute Minestrone Soup

Here's a quick version of an Italian favorite. It combines the rich flavor of fire-roasted tomatoes with fennel.

2 tablespoons extra-virgin olive oil

1 clove garlic, minced

1/4 cup chopped onion

1 slice soy "bacon" or Canadian soy "bacon," optional

1 cup chopped Swiss chard or spinach

1/2 cup cooked green beans (fresh or frozen)

1/4 cup cooked kidney beans or chick peas

1/4 cup cooked whole wheat or rice pasta (leftovers are fine)

1/4 teaspoon dried fennel seed

1/4 teaspoon Italian seasoning

14-ounce can fire-roasted tomatoes, such as Muir Glen brand

1 tablespoon dry red wine, optional

Grated Pecorino-Romano cheese for garnish

Chopped fresh basil* for garnish

| Yield: |
| 5 servings |

* Can substitute fresh basil with Pesto Sauce (page 242).

1. Heat the oil in a skillet over medium heat. Add the garlic and sauté for 1 minute, then add the onion, and continue to sauté for 4 minutes. Add the "bacon," if using, and cook another minute.

2. Stir the Swiss chard into the skillet ingredients, and sauté until wilted. Add the green beans, kidney beans, pasta, fennel, and Italian seasoning. Mix well and simmer 2 minutes before stirring in the tomatoes and wine, if using. Simmer 5 minutes, or until all of the ingredients are heated through.

3. Ladle into bowls and top with a sprinkling of grated cheese and fresh basil. Serve hot.

Mediterranean Vegetables

This is a simple, yet elegant side dish that can accompany any entrée.

Yield:
2 servings

2 medium Yukon gold potatoes, unpeeled and quartered

4 ounces fresh green beans

1 tablespoon extra-virgin olive oil

$^1/_4$ teaspoon dried oregano

$^1/_4$ teaspoon cumin

$^1/_4$ teaspoon garlic powder

Black pepper to taste

1. Preheat the oven to 450°F.

2. Toss all of the ingredients together, and place in a glass baking dish. Cover with foil and bake about 20 minutes, or until the vegetables are cooked through.

Roasted Rosemary Potatoes

Garlic and rosemary give these potatoes extraordinary flavor. Enjoy them as a side dish or snack.

Yield:
8 servings

3–4 pounds small red skin potatoes, unpeeled

$^1/_4$ cup extra-virgin olive oil

4 cloves garlic, minced

$1^1/_2$ tablespoons dried rosemary

1. Preheat the oven to 400°F.

2. Cut the potatoes in half or quarters, depending on their size, and place in a large glass baking dish. Add the olive oil and garlic. Rub the rosemary between the palms of your hands and sprinkle it on the potatoes. Mix the potatoes well.

3. Place on the middle rack of the oven and bake uncovered for 30 minutes. Transfer to the bottom rack and bake another 30 minutes, or until the potatoes are browned and cooked through.

Baked French Fries

This is a healthy, tasty alternative to French fries.

6 large red skin potatoes, unpeeled

3 tablespoons extra-virgin olive oil

One or more of the following seasonings (to taste):
garlic powder, rosemary, cajun spices, grated
Pecoroni-Romano cheese, Sun-Dried Tomato Pesto (page 243)

Yield 4 to 5 servings

1. Preheat the oven to 450°F.

2. Cut the potatoes into even strips or wedges. Place in a plastic bag along with the oil and herb(s) of choice. Close the bag and shake well to coat the potatoes. (If using pesto, reduce the amount of oil.)

3. Arrange the potatoes on a baking sheet and bake about 20 minutes, turning them at least once. Increase the oven temperature to its highest setting for another 5 to 10 minutes, or until the potatoes are crisp and brown on the outside and tender on the inside. Serve hot.

MAIN DISHES

Peasant's Secret Delight

This hearty meal is easy to make and bursting with flavor.
It is one of my family's favorites.

5 potatoes, unpeeled and cut into 2-inch cubes

2 tablespoons extra-virgin olive oil

1 cup chopped onion

$1/2$ chopped red bell pepper

$1/2$ chopped yellow bell pepper

4 soy "hot dogs" or Italian-style soy "sausage" links

1 teaspoon Old Bay seasoning

Yield:
4 servings

1. Boil the potatoes until cooked but firm. Drain and set aside.
2. Heat the oil in a skillet over medium heat. Add the onion and sauté for 3 minutes, then add the bell peppers, and continue to sauté for 5 minutes. Stir in the potatoes, and continue to cook for 5 minutes.
3. Cut the hot dogs into ½-inch slices and add to the skillet. Sprinkle with Old Bay, and cook 5 minutes, or until heated through. Serve hot.

Herbed Shrimp and Wild Rice

This meal will make you feel as if you're dining in a fine French restaurant.

Yields:
2 servings

¼ cup extra-virgin olive oil

4 cloves garlic, minced

2 tablespoons dried basil

1 tablespoon dried thyme

1 tablespoon dried parsley

12–14 medium-sized shrimp, cooked

2–3 tablespoons grated Pecorino-Romano cheese

¼ cup water

Lemon juice to taste

Sea salt to taste

Black pepper to taste

Crushed red pepper to taste

2 cups cooked wild rice

1. Heat the oil in a skillet over medium heat. Add the garlic and sauté 1 minute.
2. Place the basil, thyme, and parsley in a dish. Rub the herbs between the palms of your hands to release their flavor. Add to the skillet, and sauté about 1 minute.
3. Toss the shrimp into the skillet, and sauté about 1 minute. Add the cheese and water, and continue to cook for another minute. Add the lemon juice, salt, black pepper, and red pepper. Stir well.
4. Spoon the rice onto a serving platter and top with the shrimp mixture. Serve hot.

Lentils with Caramelized Onions

*Caramelized onions enliven the lentils and rice in this hearty entrée,
which is also great as a spread on crackers and bread.
The garnish adds a splash of color and a hint of tartness.*

1 cup uncooked lentils

6 cups water

$1/_4$ teaspoon sea salt

$1^1/_2$ cups long-grain brown rice

$2^1/_2$ teaspoons cumin

$1/_4$ cup extra-virgin olive oil

2 teaspoons minced garlic

2 large onions, sliced into rings

1 teaspoon Sucanat sugar

GARNISH

1 cup chopped tomatoes

1 cup diced green bell pepper

1 cup chopped fresh parsley

Juice of $1/_2$ lemon mixed with 2 tablespoons olive oil

Pinch sea salt

Pinch black pepper

> Yield: 4 to 5 servings

1. Place the lentils, water, and salt in a large pot. Cover and cook over medium heat for about 10 minutes. Stir in the rice, cumin, and 1 tablespoon of the oil. Cover and simmer about 30 minutes, or until the rice is cooked and the lentils are tender. Remove from stove, keep covered, and let sit 5 minutes.

2. Preheat the oven to 400°F.

3. Heat the remaining oil in a skillet over medium heat. Add the garlic, onions, and Sucanat, and sauté about 15 minutes, or until the onions are golden brown.

4. Transfer the onions to a stainless steel cookie sheet, and broil for 5 to 10 minutes, turning several times until the onions are beginning to crisp. Remove and set aside.

5. Spoon the lentils and rice into a lightly oiled glass baking dish. Spread the onions on top, and bake uncovered for 10 minutes.

6. Remove from the oven, and top with the garnish ingredients before serving. Refrigerate any leftovers for three or four days.

Portabella Mushroom Sandwich

This "steak-in-disguise" sandwich is bursting with Mediterranean flavors.

Yield:
1 sandwich

1 tablespoon extra-virgin olive oil

1 medium Portabella mushroom cap

1 small sweet onion, sliced

$1/2$ teaspoon rosemary

2 tablespoons Sun-Dried Tomato Pesto (page 243),
or 1 tablespoon eggless mayonnaise, such as Vegenaise brand

2 slices whole grain bread

1 or 2 romaine lettuce leaves

1. Heat the oil in a saucepan over medium heat. Add the mushroom cap, and sauté about 5 minutes. Add the onions and rosemary, turn the cap over, and sauté another 3 minutes.
2. Spread the pesto on one slice of bread. Top with the lettuce, mushroom, and sautéed onions. Top with the remaining slice of bread, and serve.

Mediterranean Pitza

Traditional homemade pizza is delicious but time-consuming.
This version is quick, yet tastes great!
We often enjoy it alongside 15-Minute Minestrone Soup (page247).

Yield:
2 pitzas

2 whole wheat pita breads

1 large vine-ripe tomato, sliced

$1/2$ cup Pesto Sauce (page 242)

$1/4$ cup grated Pecorino-Romano cheese

$1/4$ cup grated Manchego cheese

1. Preheat the oven to 375°F.
2. Spread the pesto sauce on each pita bread. Top with tomato slices and cheese.
3. Bake for 10 to 12 minutes. Serve hot.

Sea Breeze Smoothie

This refreshing smoothie is as delightful as a gentle sea breeze.

1 cup fresh or frozen raspberries or blueberries

1 cup soy or rice milk, or fruit juice

1 frozen banana

1 cup ice cubes

1 teaspoon raw honey

> Yield: 2 smoothies
> (10 ounces each)

1. Place all of the ingredients in a blender, and blend until smooth.

2. Pour into tall glasses and serve.

Nut-iterranean Smoothie

This nutty smoothie is a Mediterranean bonanza of flavors and chock full of healthy phytochemicals monounsaturated fats.

1 frozen banana

2–3 tablespoons almond or cashew nut butter, or all-natural peanut butter

½ cup vanilla or strawberry soy milk

1 cup ice

1 teaspoon raw honey

> Yield: 1 smoothie
> (10 ounces)

1. Place all of the ingredients in a blender, and blend until smooth.

2. Pour into a tall glass and serve.

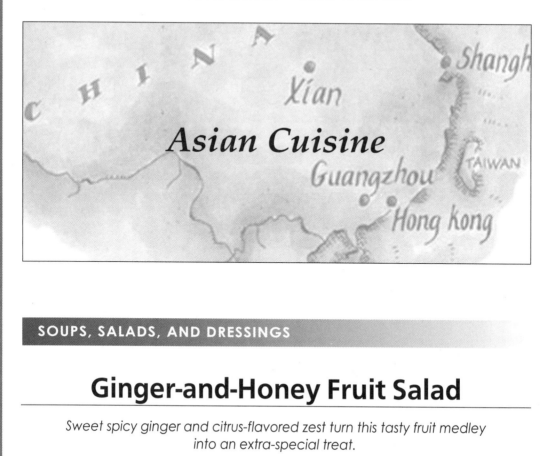

Asian Cuisine

Ginger-and-Honey Fruit Salad

Sweet spicy ginger and citrus-flavored zest turn this tasty fruit medley into an extra-special treat.

Yield:
3 servings

¼ cup raw honey
2 teaspoons minced fresh ginger
1 teaspoon lime zest
1 teaspoon orange zest
5 cups mixed fresh fruit, such as apple, pineapple, red grapes, banana, and/or kiwi
Shredded coconut for garnish

1. Combine the honey, ginger, lime zest, and orange zest in a saucepan, and place over medium heat. Simmer for 3 to 5 minutes. Remove from the heat and let cool until warm.

2. Arrange the fruit in a serving bowl, and drizzle with the honey mixture. Sprinkle with coconut and serve.

Sweet & Sour Soup

This classic soup has a slightly sweet, yet mildly spicy flavor. It reflects the healthy mindset of the Far East. For a light lunch, serve with brown rice crackers, raw cucumber slices, and carrot sticks.

1 cup cubed firm tofu

1 teaspoon cold-pressed sesame oil

1 clove minced garlic

5 medium scallions, chopped

$\frac{1}{2}$ cup chopped shiitake or other mushroom variety

1 cup chopped bok choy

2 tablespoons minced fresh ginger root

4 cups water

1 cup cooked long-grain brown rice, or brown rice noodles

Pinch cayenne pepper, optional

Yield: 3 servings

MARINADE

2 tablespoons raw honey

$\frac{1}{4}$ cup white miso, or 1 single-serve package miso soup mix

$\frac{1}{4}$ cup rice wine vinegar

2 tablespoons Bragg Liquid Aminos

1 tablespoon arrowroot powder

1. Place the tofu in a bowl. In a separate bowl, whisk together the marinade ingredients. Pour the mixture over the tofu and marinate about 20 minutes in the refrigerator.

2. Heat the oil in a large pot over medium heat. Add the garlic and sauté 1 minute, then add the scallions, and sauté 2 minutes. Toss in the mushrooms, and continue to sauté for 2 minutes. Then stir in the bok choy and ginger, and sauté another 5 minutes. Add the water and rice, and let simmer.

3. Heat a lightly oiled skillet over medium heat. Add the tofu and sear until light brown.

4. Transfer the tofu to the pot, and continue simmering until the soup has thickened. Add cayenne pepper, if desired. Serve hot.

Indian Fruit Salad

A truly delicious combination of fresh fruit and delicate spices.

Yield: 3 to 4 servings

1/4 cup water

1 tablespoon Sucanat sugar

1/2 teaspoon cinnamon

1 1/2 cups orange slices

1 1/2 cups chopped fresh or frozen peaches

1/2 cup chopped fresh pineapple

2 ripe bananas, quartered

1. Combine the water, Sucanat, and cinnamon in a saucepan, and place over medium heat. Simmer, while stirring, until the sugar is dissolved.

2. Add the fruit and toss lightly. Spoon into bowls and serve warm.

Thai Noodle Salad

This easy-to-make, colorful, and exotic salad is inspired by the unique flavors of Asia.

Yield: 6 servings

1 pound brown rice noodles

1 tablespoon extra-virgin olive oil

1/2 cup chopped red, yellow, and green bell peppers

1/2 sweet red onion, chopped

2 tablespoons toasted black sesame seeds

1 teaspoon chili oil

1 teaspoon Thai curry paste

Sea salt to taste

Black pepper to taste

1. Bring a pot of water and olive oil to boil. Add the noodles, stir, and reduce the heat to medium-low. Simmer the noodles about 10 minutes, or until cooked but not mushy. Drain and place in a bowl.

2. While the noodles are cooking, combine the remaining ingredients in a small bowl. Add to the drained noodles and toss well.

3. Refrigerate about 1 hour before serving.

Oriental Salad Dressing

*Turn ordinary vegetables into a flavorful Asian medley with this
quick and easy dressing.*

1/4 cup balsamic vinegar, or dark brown rice vinegar

3 tablespoons sesame tahini

3 tablespoons cold-pressed canola oil

2 tablespoons Sucanat sugar

1 tablespoon hot sesame oil

1 tablespoon Bragg Liquid Aminos

1/2 teaspoon fresh black pepper

Yield: About
1 cup

1. Place all of the ingredients in a blender, and blend until smooth.
2. Use immediately, or refrigerate up to 2 weeks.

MAIN DISHES AND SNACKS

Baked Wontons

*Wontons are a special snack food sold on the streets of China. Although
my family eats these wontons for breakfast, you can enjoy them any time.*

6 round wonton wrappers

1 large apple, diced

3 tablespoons unsweetened apple butter

1 tablespoon Sucanat sugar

1/4 teaspoon cinnamon

1 egg, beaten

Yield:
3 wontons

1. Preheat the oven to 350°F. Combine the apple, apple butter, Sucanat, and cinnamon in a bowl.
2. Brush three wonton wrappers with egg. Place 2 tablespoons of apple mixture in the center of each wonton. Top with a second wonton wrapper, and press the edges of the wrappers together. Brush with egg and sprinkle with Sucanat.
3. Bake about 10 minutes, or until the wontons are golden brown. Serve warm.

Shrimp Curry in a Hurry

A quick, flavorful meal that is rich in spices, yet mild enough for the "undaring" palate.

Yield:
3 servings

3 cups water

1½ cups uncooked brown rice

1 tablespoon cold-pressed peanut oil

1 cup chopped onions

¾ cup chopped red bell pepper

2 cups frozen green peas

2 tablespoons water

15 medium-sized shrimp

SAUCE

3 tablespoons cold-pressed peanut oil

4 cloves garlic, minced

2 tablespoons curry powder

2 tablespoons dried basil

1 tablespoon Bragg Liquid Aminos

2 teaspoons minced fresh ginger

½ teaspoon black pepper

1. Bring 3 cups of water to boil in a pot, and stir in the rice. Return to a boil, then reduce the heat to medium-low. Cover and simmer for 30 minutes, or until the rice is tender.

2. Heat 1 tablespoon of the oil in a wok or large deep skillet over medium heat. Add the onion and bell pepper, and sauté for 4 to 5 minutes. Transfer the mixture to a bowl, and set aside.

3. In the same wok, prepare the sauce. Heat 3 tablespoons of oil in the same wok over medium heat. Add the rest of the sauce ingredients, and stir continuously for 1 minute. Add the peas, and simmer 1 to 2 minutes. Stir in 2 tablespoons water and the sautéed bell peppers and onions. Continue simmering another minute.

4. Add the shrimp to the wok, and simmer for 2 to 3 minutes, or until it is cooked through. Add the rice, and mix all of the ingredients well. Serve hot.

Oriental Pasta

Enjoy this uniquely Asian pasta with rice crackers and green tea.

8 ounces firm tofu

3 tablespoons cold-pressed dark sesame oil

1 medium carrot, julienned

2 cups broccoli florets

1 cup sliced snow peas

1 small red pepper, julienned

3 scallions, sliced lengthwise into thin strips

1/8 teaspoon red pepper flakes, optional

8 ounces cooked brown rice noodles

Chile dipping sauce, optional

Yield:
4 servings

MARINADE

4 cloves garlic, minced

1/4 cup Bragg Liquid Aminos

1/4 cup rice vinegar

1/4 cup mirin (Chinese cooking wine)

2 tablespoons honey mustard

2 teaspoons grated fresh ginger root

1 tablespoon arrowroot or cornstarch

1. Place the tofu in a colander. Cover with a plate, and top with a heavy weight (such as a bag of beans or a gallon bottle of water). Let the tofu drain for about 15 minutes, then cut into 1-inch cubes and transfer to a bowl.

2. Combine the marinade ingredients in a bowl and whisk together well. Pour over the tofu, and marinate for 30 minutes in the refrigerator.

3. Heat 1 tablespoon of the oil in a wok or large pot over medium heat. Add the tofu and cook until golden brown, then transfer to paper towels.

4. Heat the remaining oil in the wok. Add the carrots, broccoli, snow peas, and bell peppers. Sauté 5 to10 minutes, stirring occasionally.

5. Add the scallions, tofu, and marinade. Simmer 1 or 2 minutes, or until the sauce thickens. Remove from the stove, and add the pepper flakes, if using.

6. Toss the noodles and vegetables, sprinkle with dipping sauce, and serve.

Asian Poached Salmon

This delicately seasoned Asian-inspired salmon makes a light and pleasant dish for the discerning palate. Roasted Rosemary Potatoes (page 248) and a Greek Salad (page 246) are perfect accompaniments.

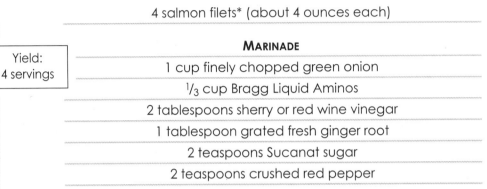

4 salmon filets* (about 4 ounces each)

MARINADE

Yield:
4 servings

1 cup finely chopped green onion

1/3 cup Bragg Liquid Aminos

2 tablespoons sherry or red wine vinegar

1 tablespoon grated fresh ginger root

2 teaspoons Sucanat sugar

2 teaspoons crushed red pepper

* Be sure to choose wild Alaskan salmon, not farm-raised or Atlantic varieties.

1. Arrange the salmon in a shallow bowl, skin side down. Mix all of the marinade ingredients together, and pour half over the fish. Refrigerate at least 15 minutes.

2. Place the fish and marinade in a skillet over medium-high heat, cover, and bring to a boil. Reduce the heat to medium-low and simmer about 5 minutes. Turn the fish over and cook another 3 to 4 minutes.

3. Transfer the fish to individual dishes, and top with the remaining marinade. Serve hot.

Skewered Singapore Tofu

This colorful, festive dish will turn an ordinary meal into a celebration.

15-ounce package 5-spice or smoked tofu, cut into 1-inch cubes

1 1/2 cups green bell pepper chunks

Yield:
5 Skewers

1 1/2 cups red bell pepper chunks

1 1/2 cups fresh pineapple chunks

1 1/2 cups onion chunks

4 cups cooked brown rice

Marinade

3 cloves garlic, minced
1/4 cup fresh lime juice
3 tablespoons Sucanat sugar
2 tablespoons fresh chopped pineapple with juice
2 tablespoons grated fresh ginger root
2 teaspoons cold-pressed canola oil
1 teaspoon curry powder
1/4 teaspoon sea salt

1. Place the tofu, bell peppers, pineapple, and onion in a glass baking dish. Mix all of the marinade ingredients together and pour over the tofu mixture. Let marinate about 20 minutes in the refrigerator.

2. Alternate the marinated ingredients onto five skewers.

3. Heat a cast iron griddle over medium heat. Add the skewers, baste with the marinade, and cook, turning when griddle marks appear on the vegetables. Serve hot over a bed of brown rice.

Curried Tofu Sandwich

A delicious (and clever) way to introduce tofu and curry to skeptics.

1 pound firm tofu
1 cup eggless mayonnaise, such as Vegenaise brand
1 1/2 teaspoons curry, or 1 teaspoon curry paste
1 1/2 tablespoons Bragg Liquid Aminos
1/4 teaspoon sea salt
1/8 teaspoon black pepper
1 cup finely diced apple
3/4 cup finely diced celery
1/2 cup chopped green onion
1 teaspoon cold-pressed canola oil
6 slices whole grain bread
1/4 cup whole wheat bread crumbs
Fresh parsley for garnish

Yield:
6 servings

1. Place the tofu in a colander. Cover with a plate, and top with a heavy weight (such as a bag of beans or a gallon bottle of water). Let the tofu drain for about 15 minutes, then cut it in half lengthwise and crumble into a bowl.

2. In another bowl, combine the mayonnaise, curry, Bragg Liquid Aminos, salt, and pepper. Fold in the apples, celery, onions, and tofu. (Add more curry if desired.)

3. Coat a cookie sheet with the oil, and arrange the bread on top.

4. Spoon the tofu-apple mixture on each slice. Top with bread crumbs and parsley.

5. Broil for 5 to 7 minutes, or until the mixture is hot and the bread is toasted. Cut each slice in half diagonally and serve.

Raspberry-Pear Breakfast Wraps

This breakfast wrap has irresistible flavors. It is a great way to start the day!

Yield: 4 wraps

2 Bosc or D'Anjou pears, sliced lengthwise

1/4 cup water

2 tablespoons maple syrup

8 ounces fresh or frozen raspberries

1/4 teaspoon cinnamon

1/2 teaspoon Sucanat sugar

4 whole wheat tortillas, such as La Tortilla Factory brand

8 ounces peach-flavored soy yogurt, such as Whole Soy brand

1. Place the pear slices, water, and maple syrup in a saucepan, and sauté over medium heat about 1 minute, or until the pears are almost tender.

2. Add the raspberries to the pears, and sprinkle with cinnamon and Sucanat. Cover and simmer about 2 minutes. Remove from the heat and let cool a bit.

3. Spread some of the warm fruit mixture on each tortilla, top with 3 to 4 tablespoons of yogurt, and roll up. Top with a dollop of yogurt and more of the fruit mixture.

4. Enjoy with a glass of fresh-squeezed orange juice.

Sesame Street Cookies

Here is something you don't often see—cookies that taste great and are actually good food you! These delicious treats are chock-full of healthy essential fats.

$1/4$ cup maple syrup

$1/4$ cup raw honey

$1/2$ cup sesame tahini

1 teaspoon natural vanilla extract, such as Frontier brand

$1/4$ cup whole wheat pastry flour

$1 1/4$ cups rolled oats

1 cup raw sunflower seeds

$1/4$ cup raw sesame seeds

Yield: About 1 dozen cookies

1. Preheat the oven to 350°F. Lightly coat a baking sheet with canola oil, and set aside.

2. Whisk together the maple syrup, honey, tahini, and vanilla in a mixing bowl. Stir in the flour, oats, and sunflower seeds. Mix well.

3. Place tablespoons of dough on the cookie sheet and flatten. Bake for 10 minutes, remove from the oven, and top with sesame seeds. Return to the oven for 5 minutes, or until the cookies are golden brown.

4. Let the cookies cool on the baking sheet for 10 minutes, before transferring them to a wire rack to finish cooling.

Conclusion

Good health is a choice. Unmistakably, the foods we choose to eat (or not eat) are an important part of this decision. Unfortunately, for millions of Americans, making the right dietary choices can be a tough and confusing process. Since the 1970s, the nation has been caught in the midst of a diet revolution in which many weight-loss plans have come and gone. Two have survived—the "high-carb, low-fat" diet, and the "low-carb, high-fat" diet. Yet, despite the persistent efforts of both diet camps, Americans continue to grow fatter.

Although the mainstream low-fat diet promoted by the USDA is trying to maintain its stronghold, the low-carb, high-fat diet is gaining ground as the more popular choice. The biggest problem, however, is that *both* diets fall short of optimal nutrition. It has been my goal through this book to make you aware of this critical truth, and offer you a health-promoting diet-and-lifestyle program that is easy, effective, and enjoyable to follow.

As you have seen, my American-MediterrAsian diet combines the best of the healthiest traditional diets of the world. Nothing like the boring "meat-and-potato" diet, or the relatively new "meat-minus-the-potato" diet, this multicultural eating strategy is flexible and diverse. It promotes delicious, satisfying meals that burst with flavor, as well as a lifestyle that encourages laughter, exercise, and social interaction. It replaces refined carbohydrates with the hardy goodness of whole grains, and radically reduces meat and poultry consumption while promoting beans, nuts, and fish. This diet also encourages the intake of fresh fruits and vegetables, uses flavorful herbs and spices to add interest to foods, and replaces hydrogenated and saturated fat with healthful oil varieties. The American-MediterrAsian lifestyle is one that promotes a cancer-free, heart-healthy, long life through an eating strategy whose health benefits have been confirmed through scientific research.

Beware the low-carb diet. It is a Trojan Horse that has passed through our gates. Without realizing its downside, millions of Americans have been celebrating the low-carb mantra with mounds of meat and other high-fat fare on their plates. At the same time, they have been restricting one of nature's greatest assets—carbs from heaven. I have pleaded with you not to be fooled by the cleverly wrapped promises offered by low-carb diets. They could be your "demise in disguise." Sure, the benefit of losing unwanted pounds in the short run while following a low-carb eating regimen is certainly inviting; however, this benefit is heavily outweighed by the diet's chronic health risks. In the long run, unsuspecting individuals will not only regain the weight they lost with a vengeance, they may also find themselves battling chronic health conditions, such as heart disease, cancer, and arthritis.

In the final analysis, I am confident that the time-proven, well-balanced, traditional plant-based diets will win over the minds and palates of the country's thinking majority. It is already beginning to happen. At the completion of this book, a growing number of restaurants and food manufacturers are starting to offer healthier choices—more than ever before. This means people are finally being given choices between carbs from heaven and those from hell. Products once primarily made with refined white flour, such as tortillas, pasta noodles, and breads, are now becoming available as 100-percent whole wheat products. Anemic white rice is no longer the only choice offered in most Chinese and Japanese restaurants— nutrient-dense, tasty brown rice is another standard option. A growing variety of vegetarian fare and health food products is making its way onto supermarket shelves, as well as restaurant menus. The pendulum is definitely swinging in favor of healthy choices.

In this book, I have offered you the eye-opening truth about diets and good health, along with all the tools you'll need to achieve a lifetime of wellness. But ultimately, the choice is yours. . . . I'm counting on you to choose wisely.

Useful Forms

Diet Diary

When following the *elimination-provocation method* or the *mono-diet challenge* to determine food sensitivities (page 87), it is important to keep track of the foods you begin reintroducing into your diet. Make copies of this seven-day diet diary and use them to maintain this record.

	Breakfast	Lunch	Dinner
SUNDAY			
MONDAY			
TUESDAY			
WEDNESDAY			
THURSDAY			
FRIDAY			
SATURDAY			

Weekly Progress Chart

Once you have made a commitment to attaining (and maintaining) a healthy lifestyle, the "7 Steps to Living Well," presented in Part 3, will help guide along you the way. After setting your personal goals, make copies of the chart below to help track your progress. A completed sample of this chart appears on page 161.

Goal	Activity	Action Steps	Feedback	Daily Points

Stool Transit Time Test

As seen in Chapter 4, regular bowel movements and short stool transit time—functions for which a high-fiber diet plays a significant role—are important for overall good health. After taking the following test, if your stool transit time is longer than twenty-four hours, you have sluggish bowel function. Following the American-MediterrAsian diet (see Chapter 13) will result in a dramatic improvement—often within seven days.

Test Procedure

1. After a bowel movement, consume either $1/2$ cup of corn or beets, or 6 black activated charcoal capsules. Record the date and time.

   Date _____   Time _____ A.M. / P.M.

2. Examine your stool and record when you first see signs of the corn, beets, or charcoal.

   Date _____   Time _____ A.M. / P.M.

3. Record when signs of the corn, beets, or charcoal are last seen in the stool.

   Date _____   Time _____ A.M. / P.M.

   TRANSIT TIME RESULTS: _____ HOURS.

References

PART 1 WHAT YOUR DOCTOR WON'T TELL YOU

Blaylock, Russell L. *Excitotoxins*. New York: Ballantine Books, 1990.

Challam, Jack. *Inflammation Syndrome*. Hoboken, NJ: John Wiley & Sons, Inc., 2003.

Hull, Janet Starr. *Sweet Poison*. Far Hills, NJ: New Horizon Press, 2001.

Lenarz, Michael. *The Chiropractic Way*. New York: Bantam Books. 2003.

Ornish, Dean. *Reversing Heart Disease*. New York: Ballantine Books, 1990.

PART 2 THE FACTS

Acheson, R. "Does Consumption of Fruit and Vegetables Protect Against Stroke?" *Lancet* 1 (1983): 1,191.

Atkins, Robert C. *Dr. Atkins' New Diet Revolution*. New York: M. Evans and Company, Inc., 2002.

Bell, IR, ML Jasnoski, J Kagan, and DS King. "Depression and allergies: survey of a nonclinical population," *Psychother Psychosom* 55 (1), (1991): 24–31.

Bennett, WG, and JJ Cerda. "Benefits of Dietary Medicine. Myth or Medicine?" *Postgrad Med* (United States) 99 (2), (1996): 153–156, 171–172.

Borghouts, LB, and HA Keizer. "Exercise and insulin sensitivity: a review," *International Journal of Sports Medicine* (Germany) 21 (1), (January 2000): 1–12.

Braly, J, and Torbert, L. *Dr. Braly's Food Allergy and Nutrition Revolution*. New Canaan, CT: Keats Publishing, Inc., 1992.

Brand-Miller, Jennie, MS Johanna, and K Foster-Powell. *Glucose Revolution Life Plan*. New York: Marlowe & Company, 2001.

Brand-Miller, R, and K Foster-Powell. "Diets with a low Glycemic index: from theory to practice," *Nutrition Today* 34 (2), (1999): 64–72.

Brody, Jane. *Jane Brody's Good Food Book: Living the High-Carbohydrate Way.* New York: Bantam Books, 1985.

Burkitt, DP, and HC Trowell. *Refined Carbohydrate Foods and Disease: Some Implications of Dietary Fiber.* London: Academic Press, 1975.

Burton Goldberg Group, The. *Alternative Medicine: The Definitive Guide.* Puyallup, WA: Future Medicine Publishing, Inc., 1993.

Chen, J, TC Campbell, J Li, and R Peto. *Diet, Lifestyle, and Mortality in China.* Oxford, England: Oxford University Press, 1990.

Cowan, CW, and PJ Watson. *The Origins of Agriculture.* Washington DC: Smithsonian Institute Press, 1992.

Day, CE. "Control of the interaction of cholesterol ester-rich lipoproteins with arterial receptors. *Atherosclerosis* 25 (Nov-Dec 1976): 199–204.

DesMaisons, Kathleen. *Potatoes Not Prozac.* New York: Fireside, 1999.

Duffy, W. *Sugar Blues.* New York: Warner Books, Inc., 1976.

Dulloo, JH, et al. "Green tea and thermogenesis: interactions between catechin-polyphenols, caffeine, and sympathetic activity," *International Journal of Obesity and Related Metabolic Disorders* 24 (February 2000): 252–258.

Dupont, Florence. *Daily Life in Ancient Rome.* Cambridge, USA: Blackwell Publishing, 1992.

Ellis, F. "Angina and Vegan Diet," *American Heart Journal* 93: 803, 1977.

Englyst, H, and J Cummings. "Digestion of the carbohydrates of the banana by the human small intestines," *American Journal of Clinical Nutrition* 44 (1986): 42–50.

Englyst, K, H Englyst, G Hudson, et al. "Rapidly available glucose in foods: an in vitro measurement that reflects the Glycemic response," *American Journal of Clinical Nutrition* 69 (1999): 448–454.

Franz, M. "Current therapies for diabetes: lifestyle modifications for diabetes management," *The Journal of Clinical Endochronology & Metabolism* 26 (3), (1997): 499–510.

Franz, M. "In defense of the American Diabetes Association's recommendations on the Glycemic index," *Nutrition Today* 34 (2), (1999): 78–81.

Gittleman, Ann Louise. *The Fat Flush Plan*. New York: McGraw-Hill, 2002.

Haenszel, W. "Studies of Japanese Migrants, Mortality from Cancer," *Journal of the National Cancer Institute* 40 (1968): 43.

Heiser, CB, Jr. *Seed to Civilization*. San Francisco: WH Freeman and Company, 1981.

Holt, SHA, JC Brand Miller, and P Petocz. "An insulin index of foods: the insulin demand generated by 1000-kj portions of common foods," *American Journal of Clinical Nutrition* 66 (1997): 1,264–1,276.

Holt, SHA, JC Brand Miller, P Petocz, and E Farmakalidis. "A satiety index of common foods," *European Journal of Clinical Nutrition* 49 (1995): 675–690.

Hunter, Beatrice Trum. "Confusing Consumers About Sugar Intake," *Consumer's Research* 78, No 1, January 1995.

Kagawa, Y. "Impact of westernization on the nutrition of Japanese: changes in physique, cancer, longevity, and centenarians," *Preventive Medicine* 7 (1978): 205–207.

Keys, Ancel. *Seven Countries: A Multivariate Analysis of Death and Coronary Heart Disease*. Cambridge, MA: Harvard University Press, 1980.

Kritchevsky, D. "Dietary Fiber and Other Dietary Factors in Hypercholesterema," *American Journal of Clinical Nutrition* 30: 979, 1977.

Lawrence, Jean. "High Fat, Low Carbs, What's the Harm?" CBS *Healthwatch*, Medscape, December 1999.

Levelle, GA, and MA Uebersax, eds. "Fundamentals of food science for the dietitian: wheat products," *Dietetic Currents* 7 (1), (1980): 1–8.

Liu, S, W Willett, M Stampfer, et al. "A prospective study of dietary Glycemic load, carbohydrate intake and risk of coronary heart disease in U.S. women," *American Journal of Clinical Nutrition* 71 (2000): 1,455–1,461.

Ludwig, D, J Majzoub, A Al-Zahrani, et al. "High Glycemic foods, overeating, and obesity," *Peds* 103 (3) (1999): 656–668.

Marmot, M. "Epidemiologic Studies of Coronary Heart Disease and Stroke in Japanese Men," *American Journal of Epidemiology* 102 (1975): 511.

McDougall, John. *McDougall's Medicine*. Chula Vista, CA: New Century Press, 1985.

Mertz, W. "Chromium in human nutrition: a review," *Journal of Nutrition* (1993): 123; 626–633.

Morris, KL, and MB Zemel. "Glycemic index, cardiovascular disease, and obesity," *Nutritional Review* 57 (9 Pt 1), (1999): 273–276.

"Nutrition recommendations and principles for people with diabetes mellitus." American Diabetes Association, position statement: http://journal.diabetes.org.

Ornish, Dean. "Effects of Stress Management Training and Dietary Changes in Treating Isochemic Heart Disease," *The Journal of the American Medical Association* 249: 54, 1983.

Peterson, TG, C Grubbs, and K Setchell. "Potential role of dietary isoflavones in the prevention of cancer," *Adv Exp Med Biol* 354 (1994): 135–147.

Pizzorno, Joseph E, *Total Wellness.* Rocklin, CA: Prima Publishing, 1996.

Robbins, John. *Diet for a New America.* Novato, CA: New World Library, 1987.

Robbins, John. *The Food Revolution.* Berkeley, CA: Conari Press, 2001.

Schoenthalen, SJ. "Diet and crime: an empirical examination of the value of nutrition in the control and treatment of incarcerated juvenile offenders," *International Journal of Biosocial Research* 4 (1983): 25–39.

Shamsuddin, AM, et al. "Ip6: A Novel Anti-Cancer Agent," *Life Sciences* 61 (1997): 343–354.

Shintani, T. *The Good Carbohydrate Revolution.* New York: Pocket Books, 2002.

Simone, CB. *Cancer and Nutrition.* Garden City Park, NY: Avery Publishing Group, 1992.

Solzman, E, and SB Roberts. "Soluble fiber and energy regulation. Current knowledge and future directions," *Adv Exp Med Bio* (United States) 427 (1997): 89–97.

Trichopoulou, A, and P Lagiou. "Healthy Traditional Mediterranean Diet: An Expression of Culture, History, and Lifestyle," *Nutrition Review* 55 (1997): 383–389.

Trowell, H. "Ischemic Heart Disease and Dietary Fiber," *American Journal of Clinical Nutrition* 25 (1972): 926.

Trowell, HD, and DP Burkitt. *Western Diseases: Their Emergence and Prevention.* Cambridge, MA: Harvard University Press, 1981.

Tsunehara, CH, DL Leonetti, and WY Fujimoto. "Diet of second-generation Japanese-American men with and without non-insulin-dependent diabetes," *American Journal of Clinical Nutrition* 52 (4), (1990): 731–738.

United States Department of Agriculture. "USDA Nutrient Database for Standard Reference," Release 12, 1999.

Vucenik, I, et al. "Comparison of Pure Inositol Hexaphosphate and High-Bran Diet in the Prevention of DMBA-Induced Rat Mammary Arcinogenesis," *Nutrition and Cancer* 28 (1987): 7–13.

Willcox, B, C Willcox, and M Suzuki. *The Okinawa Program.* New York: Three Rivers Press: 2001.

Willett, Walter C. *Eat, Drink, and Be Healthy.* New York: Fireside, 2001.

Willett, Walter C, et al. "Mediterranean Diet Pyramid: A Cultural Model for Healthy Eating," *American Journal of Clinical Nutrition* 61 (suppl), (1995): 1,402–1,406.

PART 3 LIVING WELL

American Journal of Clinical Nutrition 76 (2002): 911–922.

Appel, LJ, et al. "A Clinical Trial of the Effects of Dietary Patterns on Blood Pressure," *New England Journal of Medicine* 336 (April 17, 1997): 1,117–1,124.

Batmanghelidj, F. *Water for Health, for Healing, for Life.* New York: Warner Books, 2003.

Borghouts, LB, and HA Keizer. "Exercise and insulin sensitivity: a review," *International Journal of Sports Medicine* (Germany) 21 (1), (January 2000): 1–12.

Botting, KJ, et al. "Antimutagens in food plants eaten by Polynesians: micronutrients, phytochemicals and protection against bacterial mutagenicity of the heterocyclic amine 2-amino3-methylimidazo [4, 5-f] quinoline," *Food and Chemical Toxicology* 37 (February-March 1999): 95–103.

Clinton, SK. "Tomatoes and prostate cancer: integration of basic and clinical studies." Presented in abstract at New York Academy of Medicine, April 10, 2001.

Dulloo, JH, et al. "Green tea and thermogenesis: interactions between catechin-polyphenols, caffeine and sympathetic activity," *International Journal of Obesity and Related Metabolic Disorders* 24 (February 2000): 252–258.

Dwyer, JH, et al. "Oxygenated carotenoid lutein and progression of early atherosclerosis: the Los Angeles Atherosclerosis Study," *Circulation* 103 (June 19, 2001): 2,922–2,927.

Erasmus, Udo. *Fats That Heal, Fats That Kill.* Burnaby, BC, Canada: Alive Books, 1993.

Facchini, FS, et al. "Hyperinsulinemia: the missing link among oxidative stress and age-related diseases?" *Free Radical Biological Magazine* 12 (December 2000): 1,302–1,306.

Fujiwara, S. *Journal of Biological Chemistry* 265 (July 5, 1990): 1,333–1,337.

Gaziano, JM, et al. "A prospective study of consumption of carotenoids in fruits and vegetables, and decreased cardiovascular mortality in the elderly," *Annals of Epidemiology* 5 (July 1995), 255–260.

Iso, H, et al. "Intake of fish and omega-3 fatty acids and risk of stroke in women," *The Journal of the American Medical Association* 285 (January 17, 2001): 304–312.

Keevil, JG, et al. "Grape juice, not orange juice or grapefruit juice, inhibits human platelet aggregation," *Journal of Nutrition* 130 (January 2000): 53–56.

LeMarchand, L, et al. "Intake of specific carotenoids and lung cancer risk," *Cancer Epidemiology* 2 (May-June 1993): 183–187.

Ludwig, D, J Majzoub, A. Al-Zahrani, et al. High Glycemic foods, overeating, and obesity. *Peds* 103 (1999): 656–668.

Maas, JL, et al. "Ellagic acid, an anticarcinogen in fruits, especially in strawberries: a review," *Horticultural Science* 26 (1991): 10–14.

Michaud, DS, et al. "Intake of specific carotenoids and risk of lung cancer in 2 prospective US cohorts," *American Journal of Clinical Nutrition* 72 (October 2000): 990–997.

Mondoa, Emil I, and Mindy Kitei. *Sugars that Heal.* New York: Random House, 2001.

Morris, KL, and MB Zemel. "Glycemic index, cardiovascular disease, and obesity." *Nutritional Review* 57 (9 Part I) (1999): 273–276.

Pitchford, Paul. *Healing with Whole Foods.* Berkeley, CA: North Atlantic Books, 2002.

Proceedings of the National Academy of Sciences, vol 91, April 12, 1994.

Purba, M, et al. "Skin wrinkling: can food make a difference," *Journal of the American College of Nutrition* 20 (February 2001): 71–80.

Seibold, Ronald L., MS. *Cereal Grass. What's in It For You!: The Importance of Wheat Grass, Barley Grass, and Other Green Vegetables in the Human Diet.* Jefferson County, KS: Wilderness Community Education Foundation, 1990.

Stein, JH, et al. "Purple grape juice improves endothelial function and reduces susceptibility of LDL cholesterol to oxidation in patients with coronary artery disease," *Circulation* 100 (September 7, 1999): 1,050–1,055.

Steinmetz, KA, et al. "Vegetables, fruit, and cancer prevention: a review," *Journal of the American Dietetic Association* 96 (October 1996): 1,027–1,039.

Wang, H, et al. "Antioxidants and anti-inflammatory activities iof anthocyanins and their aglycon, cyaniding, from tart cherries," *Journal of Nutritional Products* 62 (February 1999): 294–296.

Wang, H, et al. "Antioxidants polyphenols from tart cherries (*Prunus cerasus*)," Journal of Agriculture and Food Chemistry 47 (March 1999): 840–844.

Wilson, T, et al. "Cranberry extract inhibits low density lipoprotein oxidation," *Life Sciences* 62 (1998): PL 381–386.

Zhang, T, et al. "Anticarcinogenic activities of sulforaphane and structurally related synthetic norbornyl isothiocyanates," *Proceedings of the National Academy of Sciences* 91 (April 12, 1994): 3,147–3,150.

Index

ACS. *See* American Cancer Society.
ADA. *See* American Diabetic Association.
Adaptive phase of hidden food
  allergies, 84
Adaptogens, 179
ADD. *See* Attention deficit disorder.
Adrenal glands, 71–72
Adrenaline, 206
Agatston, Arthur, 77
Agriculture, Department of.
    See Department of Agriculture.
Alarm phase of hidden food allergies, 81
Allen, Woody, 96, 97
Allergies, food. *See* Food allergies.
Alpha-linolenic acid, 176
AMA. *See* American Medical
  Association.
American Cancer Society, 11, 117
American Diabetic Association, 64, 112
American Dietetic Association, 11
American Heart Association, 11, 15, 16,
  23, 56, 92, 93, 110, 139, 142, 151, 168
American Institute for Cancer Research,
  117
American Journal of Cardiology, 110
American Journal of Clinical Nutrition, 102
American Kidney Fund, 150
American Medical Association, 25, 26,
  27, 28
American-MediterrAsian diet,
  about, 211–217

shopping list for, 218–220
recipes for, 227–263
American-MediterrAsian Diet and
  Lifestyle Pyramid, 216
Anderson, James, 64, 65, 145
Angell, Marcia, 14
Anthocyanins, 164
Antigens, 84
Antioxidants
  and carbohydrates from
    heaven, 54–55
  as defense against aging, 53
  as disease fighters, 53
  and inflammation, 22, 23
  and Ip6 factor, 121
"Apple Pie" Go-Go Juice, 183
Apple-shaped figures, 112–113
Asian diet, 40, 103, 111, 124, 125,
  133–136
Asian Food Pyramid, 133
Asian Poached Salmon, 260
Ask-Upmark, Erik, 172
Aspartame, 17–19
Atkins, Robert, 23, 65, 77, 90, 144, 145,
  146, 148, 149, 194
Atkins' Diet, 23, 65, 77, 91, 92, 97, 145,
  146, 149–152, 191, 198
Atkins' Health and Medical Information
  Services, 152
Atkins' Physician Council, 92
Attention deficit disorder, 73

Baked French Fries, 249

Baked Wontons, 257

Ballantyne, Christie, 112

Banting, William, 143, 144

Barley grass, 179, 180

Baylor College of Medicine, 112, 191

Bee pollen, 172–173

Berry Delicious Smoothie, 237

Best Burrito Ever, 232

Beta-carotene, 164

Beta-sistosterol, 177

Bile, 199

Biological stress syndrome, 81

Blaylock, R., 18

Block, Gladys, 151

Blood sugar, low. *See* Hypoglycemia.

Blood sugar levels, 61–62, 70–71.
    See also Hypoglycemia.

Blueberry Breakfast Crisp, 227

Blueberry Go-Go Smoothie, 183

Braly, James, 68, 80

Bran (seed), 50, 51

Bravata, Dena, 91

Bread, history of, 39–40

Breakfast, Frisco Bay, 228

Breakfast Burrito, 229

Breakfast Wraps, Raspberry-Pear, 262

Brigham and Women's Hospital, 21

Brown adipose tissue. *See* Brown fat.

Brown fat, 205

Brown University, 148

Bruschetta, 241

Buerkitt, Dennis, 55–56, 57

Burrito, Best, Ever, 232

Burrito, Breakfast, 229

Cabbage Soup diet, 191

Caesar Salad, 245

Caesar Salad Dressing, 245

California, University of, Berkeley, 152

California, University of, Davis, 102

California, University of, San Francisco,
    110, 116

California "Dagwood" Sandwich, 234

Campbell, Colin, 136

Campesterol, 177

Cancer
    and diet, 116–122
    and saturated fat, 145, 146, 147
    statistics for, 116
    and whole grains, 119–120

Caramelized Onions, Lentils with, 251

Carbohydrates
    and American-MediterrAsian diet,
      212–213, 217
    and Asian diet, 134
    anatomy of, 50
    and behavioral disorders, 67
    and blood sugar levels, 61, 70–71, 78
    complex, 47, 50
    digestible, 45
    and effect on cancer, 116–122
    and effect on heart health,
      109–116, 119
    and effect on fullness, 106
    as energy source, 45
    formation of, 45
    as foundation for wellness, 166–167
    indigestible, 45–46
    and inflammation, 21–22
    and Latin American diet, 131
    and low-carb diets, 138
    and Mediterranean diet, 138
    metabolism of, 62–63
    simple, 47
    sources of, 46, 46
    and standard American diet, 127
    tips when purchasing, 42–43
    See also Carbohydrates, refined;
      Carbohydrates from heaven;
      Carbohydrates from hell; Diets,
      weight-loss; Glycemic index;
      Power carbs.

Carbohydrates, refined
    and effect on blood sugar, 51, 61–62,
      106–107

and hyperactivity
and insulin resistance, 63–64
and Syndrome X, 41
See also Carbohydrates from hell.
Carbohydrates from heaven, 46–47
anatomy of, 50
as cancer preventive, 116–122
as diet of ancestors, 96
and effect on fullness, 106
and effect on heart health, 116
and effect on insulin and blood
sugar, 62, 70, 78, 106–107
listing of, 48
as vitamin and mineral source,
52–53, 118–120
Carbohydrates from hell, 46
and effect on adrenal glands, 71–72
and effect on insulin and blood
sugar, 61–62, 70, 78, 106–107
and fructose, 102
listing of, 49
tips when eating, 121–122
See also Carbohydrates, refined.
Cardiomyopathy, 23
Cardiovascular disease. *See* Heart
disease.
Carotenoids, 164
CDC. *See* Centers for Disease
Control.
Celebrex, 179
Celiac disease, 78
Celiac Foundation, 79
Cell membrane, 168
Cells, about, 53, 168
Centers for Disease Control, 89
Cereal, Couscous Breakfast, 239
Cereal grass, 179, 180–181
Charlamagne, 175
Chili "non" Carne, Fiesta, 235
Chipotle Mayonnaise, 232
Chiropractic health care, 28–31
Chiropractic physicians, 27–31
nutritional training of, 30

and treatment from AMA, 27–28
Chlorophyll, 181
Cholesterol
effects of fiber on, 115–116
HDL, 115
LDL, 110, 114, 115, 168
and the liver, 114–115
as risk factor for heart attack, 20
as risk factor for stroke, 20
and statin drugs, 115–116
Chromium, 52–53, 176
Chromium picolinate, 66
Cleveland Clinic, 21
Conway, Leo, 173
Cookies, Sesame Street, 263
Cooler, Lemon-Watermelon, 238
Corn syrup, high fructose, 102
Cornell-China Oxford Project, 136
Cornell University, 133, 136
Cortisol, 206
Couscous Breakfast Cereal, 239
Crawford, Paul, 150
C-Reactive protein, 21, 150
Crisp, Blueberry Breakfast, 227
Critser, Greg, 102
Curried Tofu Sandwich, 261–262
Curry in a Hurry, Shrimp, 258
Cyanogenic glycosides, 176

"Dagwood" Sandwich, California, 234
Dairy products
and Asian diet, 134, 135
and Latin American diet, 131
and Mediterranean diet, 138
and standard American diet, 127–128
Damnacanthal, 179
DDT, 19–20
Delayed food allergies, 79–80
Delight, Peasant's Secret, 249–250
Department of Agriculture, 68, 89, 96,
117, 164, 172, 200. *See also* Food
Guide Pyramid, USDA; Standard
American diet.

Department of Health and Human
    Services, 18, 117
Despres, Jean-Pierre, 66
Diabetes, type I, 64, 66
Diabetes, type II, 63, 103
DiAngelis, D., 12
Diet Diary form, 268
Diets, weight-loss
    Atkins, 23, 65, 77, 91, 92, 93, 97
    calorie comparison for, 93
    debate over, 88–89
    high-fat, 97
    low-carb, 9–11, 77–78, 89, 90–93
    low-fat, 89
    obsession with, 90
    plant-based, 103, 110, 111, 124
    South Beach, 77, 91, 97,
    statistics for, 77
    Sugar Busters, 97
    traditional versus "westernized,"
        40–41
    Zone, 77, 89, 91
    See also American-MediterrAsian
        diet; Asian diet; Latin American
        diet; Low-Carb, High-Protein diet;
        Standard American diet.
Dip, Mediterranean Hummus, 242
Dis-ease, 156–157
Dr. Atkins' Diet Revolution (Atkins),
    77, 144
Dr. Atkins' New Diet Revolution (Atkins),
    77, 90, 93
Dr. Braly's Food Allergy and Nutrition
    Revolution (Braly), 80
Dressing, Caesar Salad, 245
Dressing, Oriental Salad, 257
Dressing, South-of-the-Border, 230
Duke University, 198
Duke University Medical School, 146

Eckel, Robert, 93, 151
EFAs. See Essential fats.
Eggs, organic, 220

Eggs, Herbed Scrambled, 240
Eisenhower, Dwight D., 30
Elimination-provocation method for
    determining allergies, 87
ELISA food allergy blood test, 68, 74, 87,
    92, 167, 197, 198
Ellagic acid, 164
Elsas, Louis, 18
Emmer, 38
Emory Medical School, 18
Endorphins, 207
Endosperm (seed), 50, 51
Enkalphin hormones, 207
Equal, 17, 18
Eskimos, diet of, 148, 149
Essential fats, 169, 170, 204. See also Fat,
    dietary; Omega-3 fats; Omega-6
    fats.
Essential fatty acid deficiency, 170
Essential fatty acids. See Essential fats.
Excitotoxins: the Taste that Kills
    (Blaylock), 18
Exercise
    and daily routine, 186
    and effect on insulin resistance,
        65–66
    and games for getting energized,
        186–188
    and "wellness," 185
Exhaustive phase of hidden food
    allergies, 84

Fairfield, Kathleen, 25, 26
Fajita without the "Meata," 233
Fast-food American diet. See Standard
    American diet.
Fast Food Nation (Schlosser), 183
Fat, dietary
    and American-MediterrAsian
        diet, 213
    and Asian diet, 134
    and Latin American diet, 131
    and low-carb, high-protein diet, 145

and Mediterranean diet, 138–139
phony, 16, 85, 87, 198
and standard American diet, 128
See also Essential fats; Hydrogenated
fats and oils; Monounsaturated fat,
Omega 3 fats; Omega-6 fats;
Polyunsaturated fat; Saturated fat.
Fat Land (Critser), 102
Fattoush Salad with Whole Wheat Pitas,
243–244
FDA. *See* Food and Drug Administration.
Federal Office of Alternative Medicine,
27, 29
Fenugreek seeds, 66
Fiber, dietary
as appetite suppressant, 60
as breast cancer preventive, 120–121
as calorie blocker, 96
digestible, 45
and feeling of fullness, 106
and fiber theory of disease,
and food sources, 58–59
and glycemic index, 100
and good health, 46, 47, 50, 55
health problems linked to low, 55,
56, 57
indigestible, 45–46
and lowering cholesterol, 115–116
and stool transit time, 55, 56
water-soluble, 115, 116
for weight loss, 195
See also High complex-fiber diet.
Fiber theory of disease, 55–56
Fiesta Chili "non" Carne, 235
15-Minute Minestrone Soup, 247
"Fight or flight" response, 71–72
Fish, safety guidelines for, 140–141
Flax flour, 116
Flaxative, 176
Flaxseed oil, 116
Flaxseeds, 116, 175–177
Fleming, Richard M., 150
Fleming Heart & Health Institute, 150

Fletcher, Robert, 25, 26
Food allergies, 68, 74, 78–88, 196–197
delayed, 79–80
and gluten sensitivity, 78–79
and leaky gut syndrome, 79
phases of, 81, 84–85
and phony fat, 85, 87
questionnaire for, 82–83
symptoms of, 80–81
tests for determining, 87
Food and Drug Administration, 18, 19,
69
Food Guide Pyramid, USDA, 123–124,
126–129
Food pyramids. *See* American-
MediterrAsian Diet and Lifestyle
Pyramid; Asian Food
Pyramid; Food Guide Pyramid,
USDA; Latin American Food
Pyramid; Low- Carb, High-Protein
Food Pyramid; Mediterranean
Food Pyramid.
Food Revolution, The (Robbins), 151
Foreyr, John, 191
Four Basic Food Groups, 123, 129
Free radicals
and heart disease, 22
and polyunsaturated fat, 169
as threat to cells, 54–55
French Fries, Baked, 249
Frisco Bay Breakfast, 228
Fruit & Granola Parfait, 240
Fruit Salad, Ginger-and-Honey, 254
Fruit Salad, Indian, 256
Fucose, 174
Functional food, 181

Galactose, 174
Gamma-linolenic acid, 181, 204–205
Gaynor, Mitchell, 117
G.D. Searle, 17
Germ (seed), 50, 51
Getzendanner, Susan, 27

Ginger-and-Honey Fruit Salad, 254
GLA. *See* Gamma-linolenic acid.
Glucose, 61, 62, 63, 174, 206
Glucose Revolution, The, 97
Glucose tolerance test, 71
Gluten sensitivity, 78–79
Glycemic index, 62, 96–106
    about, 96–98
    facts and flaws, 98–99, 100, 101
    and Pima paradox, 103–104
    sample food table, 99
    See also Insulin Score; Satiety Index.
Glycogen, 62
Glyconutrients, 174–175
Grains, history of, 38–41
Greek Salad, 246
Green tea, 134, 135, 136
Guar gum, 66

Hagiwara, Y., 180
Harper's Biochemistry, 174
Harvard Medical School, 15, 20, 21, 25,
    52, 116, 163, 205
Harvard Medical School of Psychiatry, 68
Harvard School of Public Health, 52, 123,
    124, 133
Harvard University, 41
Harvey, William, 143
Havel, Peter, 102
HCF diet. *See* High complex-fiber diet.
Health and Human Services, Department
    of. *See* Department of Health and
    Human Services.
Health News Analyzer, 9
Healthy Indulgences chart, 221–223
Heart attacks. *See* Heart disease.
Heart disease
    and apple-shaped figure, 112–113
    and diet, 109–114
    and healthy fats, 114
    and inflammation, 20–21
    and link to diabetes, 41
    and link to Syndrome X, 112

and plant-based diet, 109, 110–111
and saturated fat and cholesterol,
    114, 145
statistics for, 109, 111
Heber, David, 119
Heimowitz, Colette, 152
Heinicke, Ralph, 178
Hemus, Peter, 172
Herbed Scrambled Eggs, 240
Herbed Shrimp and Wild Rice, 250
High complex-fiber diet, 64–65
Hippocrates, 175
Holt, Susanna, 105
Homocysteine, 26, 164
Hull (seed), 50, 51
Hummus Dip, Mediterranean, 242
Hydrogenated fats and oils, 15–16, 17, 19,
    111, 128, 168. *See also* Fat, dietary.
Hydrogenation, 168
Hypoglycemia, 63, 70, 71, 72–73, 199

I Love Lucy, 200
IgG mediated allergy, 80
Immediate-onset allergic reactions, 79
Indian Fruit Salad, 256
Indiana, University of, 194
Indole-3-carbonol, 165
Industrial Revolution, 40
Inflammation
    and adrenal glands, 71
    and carbohydrates, 21–22
    causes of, 20, 22, 23, 24–25
    and heart disease, 20–21
    and low-carb diets, 23
    and normal body function, 22
    ways to eliminate, 212
Inflammatory prostaglandins, 196
Insulin, 47, 52, 62, 63, 78, 106–107, 144.
    See also Hypoglycemia; Insulin
    resistance; Insulin Score;
    Syndrome X.
Insulin-dependent diabetes. *See* Diabetes,
    type I.

Insulin resistance, 63–64, 65, 70, 112
Insulin Score, 106
Intestines
    function of, 197–199
    ways to maintain healthy, 199–201
Ip6 factor, 121
Isoflavones, 119
I3C. *See* Indole-3-carbonal.

JAMA. *See Journal of the American Medical Association, The.*
Japanese Ministry of Health, 136
Johns Hopkins Medical School, 165, 178
Jones, Wayne, 27, 29, 30
Journal of Agriculture Research, 179
Journal of the American Medical Association, The, 9, 12, 14, 25, 26, 91, 116
Journal of Kidney Disorders, 150
Journal of the National Cancer Institute, The, 172

Kentucky, University of, Metabolic Center, 145
Ketosis, 149–150, 151
Keys, Ansel, 15
Kneipp, Father Sebastian, 155

Lactose, 46
Laim, Chiu Nan, 179
Lancet, The, 196
Lasagna, Mexican, 236
Latin American diet, 40, 124, 125, 130–132
Laughter
    importance of for wellness, 188–190
    prescription for, 189
Laval University Hospital, 66
Leaky gut syndrome, 79
Leander, Gosta, 172
Lee, Phillip, 116
Lemon-Watermelon Cooler, 238
Lentils with Caramelized Onions, 251

Leptin, 102, 207
Lignans, 116, 119, 175–176
Lipid Research Center at Laval University Hospital, 66
Lipitor, 115
Lipofuscin, 55
Lipotropic herbs, 201
Liver
    function of, 197–199
    ways to maintain healthy, 199–201
Loma Linda University, 147
Lonsdale, Derick, 68
Low-carb, high-protein diet, 125, 143–152, 199. *See also* Atkins' Diet.
Low-Carb, High-Protein Food Pyramid, 125, 130
Low-carb diets. *See* Diet, low-carb; Low-carb, high-protein diet.
Lycopene, 139, 163–164
Lyon Study, 139, 140, 142

Malathion, 180
Mannose, 174
Maryland, University of, 121
Maryland, University of, School of Medicine, 206
Massachusetts Institute of Technology, 19
Mayo Clinic, 203
Mayonnaise, Chipotle, 232
McCully, K., 26
McNab, Tom, 173
Medical University of Mississippi, 18
Mediterranean diet, 40, 111, 124, 125, 137–142, 169, 205, 206
Mediterranean Food Pyramid, 137
Mediterranean Hummus Dip, 242
Mediterranean Pitza, 252
Mediterranean Vegetables, 248
Mercury levels in fish, 140–141
Methodist DeBakey Heart Center, 112
Methylphenidate. *See* Ritalin.
Mexican Lasagna, 236
Mexican Taco Salad, 230

Michigan, University of, Human Nutrition Program, 37
Minestrone Soup, 15-Minute, 247
Mississippi, Medical University of. *See* Medical University of Mississippi.
MIT. *See* Massachusetts Institute of Technology.
Mono-diet challenge for determining allergies, 87
Monounsaturated fat, 111, 114–115, 169, 204. *See also* Fat, dietary.
Montreal University of, 205
Morinda citrifolia. See Tahitian noni fruit.
Mucopolysaccharides, 181
MUFAs. *See* Monounsaturated fat.

N-acetyleuraminic acid, 175
N-acetylgalactoseamine, 174
N-acetylglucosamone, 174
Nass, Meryl, 9
National Cancer Institute, 165
National Dairy Council, 135, 136
National Health and Nutrition Examination Survey, 129
National Institutes of Health, 27, 29
National Research Council, 69
National Weight Control Registry, 148
NCI. *See* National Cancer Institute.
Nerve sheath, 168
New England Journal of Medicine, The, 14, 15, 69–70, 147, 197
New York Time, The, 92
Newsweek, 110, 117, 119
NIH. *See* National Institutes of Health.
Noninsulin-dependent diabetes. *See* Diabetes, type II.
Noodle Salad, Thai, 256
Nurses Health Study, 15, 52, 63, 116
Nut-iterranean Smoothie, 253
NutraSweet, 17–19, 20

OAM. *See* Federal Office of Alternative Medicine.

Oat Pancakes, 229
Oil & Vinegar Salad, Quick, 244
Okinawa Centenarian Study, 136
Oldways International, 124, 133
Olive oil, 205–206
Olney, John, 18
Omega-3 fats, 66, 111, 114–115, 169–171, 176, 204, 205. *See also* Fat, dietary.
Omega-6 fats, 169–171, 204, 205. *See also* Fat, dietary.
Oolong tea, 134, 135, 136
Opioid-morphine drugs, 196
Oriental Pasta, 259
Oriental Salad Dressing, 257
Ornish, Dean, 32, 106, 110, 198

Paffenbarger, Ralph S., 65–66
Pancakes, Oat, 229
Parfait, Fruit & Granola, 240
Passwater, Richard, 22
Pasta, Oriental, 259
Peasant's Secret Delight, 249–250
Peeke, Pamela, 206
Peristalsis, 200
Pesto, Sun-Dried Tomato, 243
Pesto Sauce, 242
P4D1, 180–181
PGs. *See* Prostaglandins.
Philadelphia Veterans Administration Hospital, 146
Phony fat, 16, 85, 87, 198
Phytic acid. *See* Ip6 factor.
Phytochemicals, 118–120
Pima Indians, 103–104, 132
Pima paradox, 103–104, 132
Piña Colada Smoothie, 238
Pitza, Mediterranean, 252
"Plastic foods," 16
Poached Salmon, Asian, 260
Polyunsaturated fat, 111, 168–169, 181. *See also* Fat, dietary.
Portabella Mushroom Sandwich, 252
Potatoes, Roasted Rosemary, 248

Power carbs, 171–184
Pravachol, 115
Prostaglandins, 24–25, 204–205
Protein
    and American-MediterrAsian diet,
      213, 217
    and Asian diet, 134
    dietary importance of, 144
    and Latin American diet, 131
    and low-carb, high-protein diet, 144
    and Mediterranean diet, 138
    and standard American diet, 127
Proxeronine, 178
Prudent diet, 139, 142

Quick Oil & Vinegar Salad, 244

Raglin, Jack, 194
Randolph, Theron, 80
Raspberry-Pear Breakfast Wraps, 262
Reaven, Gerald, 41, 112
Refining process of grains, 51
Rennie, Drummond, 14
Resveratrol, 165
Reversing Heart Disease (Ornish), 110
Rhammose, 181
Ridker, Paul, 20, 21
Ritalin, 73, 74
Roasted Rosemary Potatoes, 248
Robbins, John, 151
Robinson, William, 172–173
Rosemary Potatoes, Roasted, 248
Royal Jelly, 173
Royalisin, 173

Salad, Caesar
Salad, Fattoush, with Whole Wheat
    Pitas, 243–244
Salad, Ginger-and-Honey Fruit, 254
Salad, Greek, 246
Salad, Indian Fruit, 256
Salad, Mexican Taco, 230
Salad, Quick Oil & Vinegar, 244

Salad, Thai Noodle, 256
Salad, West Coast Salmon, 231
Salad Dressing, Caesar, 245
Salad Dressing, Oriental, 257
Salmon, Asian Poached, 260
Salmon Salad, West Coast, 231
Samaha, Frederick, 146–147
Sandwich, California "Dagwood," 234
Sandwich, Curried Tofu, 261–262
Sandwich, Portabella Mushroom, 252
Satiety Index, 104–106
Saturated fat
    about, 168
    and cancer, 145, 146, 147
    and heart disease, 151
    and standard American diet, 111
    and Syndrome X, 41
    See also Fat, dietary.
Sauce, Pesto, 242
Schlosser, Eric, 183
Science Magazine, 174
Scientific American, 174
Scopoletin, 178–179
Scrambled Eggs, Herbed, 240
Scratch test, skin. *See* Skin scratch test.
Sea Breeze Smoothie, 253
Searle, G.D. *See* G.D. Searle.
Sears, Barry, 77, 89, 91
Secret Delight, Peasant's, 249–250
Selye, Hans, 81
Sesame Street Cookies, 263
Seven Country Study, 139, 140, 141–142
7-Day American-MediterrAsian Menu
    Plan, 226
7-Step Knockout Weight-Loss Plan,
    191–208
7 Steps to Living Well, 157–162, 163–184,
    185–190
Shamberger, Raymond, 68
Shrimp, Herbed, and Wild Rice, 250
Shrimp Curry in a Hurry, 258
SI. *See* Satiety Index.
Singapore Tofu, Skewered, 260–261

Skewered Singapore Tofu, 260–261
Skin scratch test, 79
Slatter, James, 17
Sleep deprivation, 207
Sleeper, 96
Sloppy Joes, 234
Smoothie, Blueberry Go-Go, 183
Smoothie, Nut-iterranean, 253
Smoothie, Sea Breeze, 253
SOD. *See* Superoxide dismutase.
Solomon, Neil, 178
Soup, 15-Minute Minestrone, 247
Soup, Sweet & Sour, 255
South Beach Diet, 91, 97, 144
South Beach Diet, The (Agatston), 77
South-of-the-Border Dressing, 230–231
Spirulina, 181, 183
Standard American diet, 111, 126–129,
    191, 205. *See also* Food Guide
    Pyramid, USDA.
Stanford University, 41
Stanford University School of Medicine,
    66, 91
Statin drugs, 115–116
Sterols, 177
Stigmasterol, 177
Stillman Diet, 144
Stone-Age diet, 37
Stool transit time, 56, 57, 270
Strang-Cornell Cancer Prevention
    Center, 117
Stress, 201
Stress hormones, 206–207
Stress-management skills, 201
Stress without Distress (Selye), 81
Sugar
    consumption of, 69
    harmful effects of, 69–71
Sugar Blues (Duffy), 69
Sugar Busters, 97
Sugar Busters Diet, 97
Sugars, essential.
    See Glyconutrients.

Sulpheraphane, 201
Sun-Dried Tomato Pesto, 243
Superoxide dismutase, 180–181
Sweet & Sour Soup, 255
Sweeteners, artificial, 17–19, 20
"Sweetgate," 20
Syndrome X, 41, 64, 70, 111–114

Taco Salad, Mexican, 230
Tahitian noni fruit, 177
Tahitian noni juice, 177–179
Tahitian Noni Juice: How Much, How Often,
    For What (Solomon), 178
Texas, University of, Medical Center, 179
Texas, University of, Southwestern, 150
Thai Noodle Salad, 256
Thalidomide, 19
Thermogenesis, 204
Tofu Sandwich, Curried, 261–262
Tofu, Skewered Singapore, 260–261
Topol, Eric, 21
Trager, Stuart, 92
Trans fats. *See* Hydrogenated fats
    and oils.
Turmeric, 201

United States Department of Agriculture.
    See Department of Agriculture.
United States Department of Health and
    Human Services. *See* Department of
    Health and Human Services.
United States Food and Drug
    Administration. *See* Food and Drug
    Administration.
University of California, Berkeley. *See*
    California, University of, Berkeley.
University of California, Davis. *See*
    California, University of, Davis.
University of California, San Francisco.
    See California, University of, San
    Francisco.
University Hospital of London,
    Ontario, 195

University of Indiana. *See* Indiana, University of.

University of Kentucky Medical School. *See* Kentucky, University of, Medical School.

University of Kentucky Metabolic Center. *See* Kentucky, University of, Metabolic Center.

University of Maryland. *See* Maryland, University of.

University of Maryland School of Medicine. *See* Maryland, University of, School of Medicine.

University of Michigan Human Nutrition Program. *See* Michigan, University of, Human Nutrition Program.

University of Montreal. *See* Montreal, University of.

University of Texas, Southwestern. *See* Texas, University of, Southwestern.

University of Texas Medical Center. *See* Texas, University of, Medical Center.

University of Vienna. *See* Vienna, University of.

University of Wisconsin Medical School. *See* Wisconsin, University of, Medical School.

Uric acid, 145

USDA. *See* Department of Agriculture.

USDA Food Guide Pyramid. *See* Food Guide Pyramid, USDA.

Vegetables, Mediterranean, 248

Vienna, University of, 172

Villi, 62

Vioxx, 179

Vitamin B
for brain and nervous system functioning, 67–68

and role in reducing homocysteine, 26

"Vitamin HaHa," 188, 189

Vitamins
and effect on free radicals, 55
and role in good health, 25–27, 183
and effect on insulin, 66

Washington University, 18

Water, importance of, 202–203

Weekly Progress Chart, 161, 2669

Wellness
definition of, 155–156
7 Steps to, 157–162, 163–184, 185–190

Wellness buddy, 193–194

Wellness coach, 158–159

West Coast Salmon Salad, 231

Western Diseases: Their Emergence and Prevention (Buerkitt), 56

Wheat grass, 179, 180

Wild Rice, Herbed Shrimp and, 250

Wing, Rena, 148

Wisconsin, University of, Medical School, 165

WHO. *See* World Health Organization.

"Whoops" factor, 19–20

Willett, Walter, 123, 124

Wontons, Baked, 257

World Health Organization, 10, 124

Wraps, Raspberry-Pear Breakfast, 262

Wurtman, R., 19

Xeronine, 178

Xylose, 174

Yale University, 91

Zocor, 115

Zone, The (Sears), 77, 91

Zone Diet, 89, 144

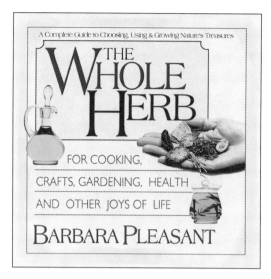

THE WHOLE HERB
For Cooking, Crafts, Gardening, Health, and Other Joys of Life
Barbara Pleasant

Herbs are nature's pure and precious gifts. They provide sustenance for both our bodies and our souls. They have been our medicine and our food. Their fragrance and beauty have warmed our hearts and delighted our senses.

The Whole Herb is a complete, practical, and easy-to-follow guide to the many uses of these wonderful treasures of the earth. It presents their fascinating history, as well as their many uses, including herbs and health, herbs and cooking, herbs around the house, and herbs in the garden. A comprehensive A-to-Z reference profiles over fifty commonly used and affordable herb varieties. Each entry provides specific information on the herb's background, benefits, and uses, along with helpful buying guides, growing instructions, preservation methods, and safety information.

Whether you want to use herbs to create better health, better meals, unforgettable fragrances, impressive crafts, or a beautiful garden, *The Whole Herb* is here to help.

$14.95 US / $22.50 CAN • 228 pages • 7.5 x 7.5-inch paperback • 2-Color • Reference/Herbs • ISBN 0-7570-0080-0

GOING WILD IN THE KITCHEN
The Fresh & Sassy Tastes of Vegetarian Cooking
Leslie Cerier

Going Wild in the Kitchen is the first comprehensive global vegetarian cookbook to go beyond the standard organic beans, grains, and vegetables. In addition to providing helpful cooking tips and techniques, the book contains over 200 kitchen-tested recipes for healthful, taste-tempting dishes—creative masterpieces that contain such unique ingredients as edible flowers; sea vegetables; wild mushrooms, berries, and herbs; and goat and sheep cheeses. It encourages the creative side of novice and seasoned cooks alike, prompting them to follow their instincts and "go wild" in the kitchen by adding, changing, or substituting ingredients in existing recipes. To help, a wealth of suggestions is found throughout. Beautiful color photographs and a helpful resource list for finding organic foods complete this user-friendly cookbook.

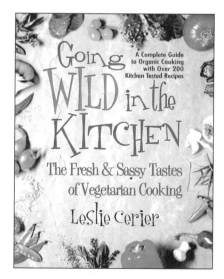

Going Wild in the Kitchen is both a unique cookbook and a recipe for inspiration. So let yourself go! Excite your palate with this treasure-trove of unique, healthy, and taste-tempting recipe creations.

$16.95 US / $25.50 CAN • 224 pages • 7.5 x 9-inch paperback • 2-Color • Full-color photos • Cooking/Vegetarian • ISBN 0-7570-0091-6

KITCHEN QUICKIES
Great, Satisfying Meals in Minutes
Marie Caratozzolo and Joanne Abrams

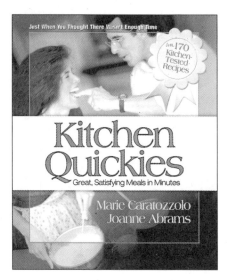

Ever feel that there aren't enough hours in the day to enjoy life's pleasures—simple or otherwise? Whether you're dealing with problems on the job, chasing after kids on the home front, or simply running from errand to errand, the evening probably finds you longing for a great meal, but with neither the time nor the desire to prepare one.

Kitchen Quickies offers a solution. Virtually all of its over 170 kitchen-tested recipes—yes, really kitchen tested—call for a maximum of only five main ingredients other than kitchen staples, and each dish takes just minutes to prepare! Imagine being able to whip up dishes like Southwestern Tortilla Pizzas, Super Salmon Burgers, and Tuscan-Style Fusilli—in no time flat! As a bonus, these delicious dishes are actually good for you—low in fat and high in nutrients!

So the next time you think that there's simply no time to cook a great meal, pick up *Kitchen Quickies.* Who knows? You may even have time for a few "quickies" of your own.

$14.95 US / $22.50 CAN • 240 pages • 7.5 x 9-inch quality paperback • Full-color photos • Cooking • ISBN 0-7570-0085-1

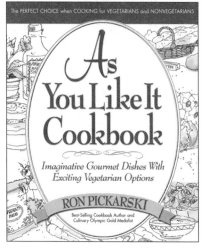

AS YOU LIKE IT COOKBOOK
Imaginative Gourmet Dishes with Exciting Vegetarian Options
Ron Pickarski

When it comes to food, we certainly like to have it our way. However, catering to individual tastes can pose quite a challenge for the cook. The *As You Like It Cookbook* is designed to help you meet the challenge of cooking for both vegetarians and nonvegetarians alike. It offers over 170 great-tasting dishes that cater to a broad range of tastes. Many of the easy-to-follow recipes are vegetarian—and offer ingredient alternatives for meat eaters. Conversely, recipes that include meat, poultry, or fish offer nonmeat ingredient options. Furthermore, if the recipe includes eggs or dairy products, a vegan alternative is provided. This book has it all—delicious breakfast favorites, satisfying soups and sandwiches, mouth-watering entrées, and delectable desserts.

With one or two simple ingredient substitutions, the *As You Like It Cookbook* will show you how easy it is to transform satisfying meat dishes into delectable meatless fare, and vegetarian dishes into meat-lover's choices.

$16.95 US / $25.50 CAN • 216 pages • 7.5 x 9-inch quality paperback • Full-color photos • Cooking • ISBN 0-7570-0013-4

For more information about our books, visit our website at www.squareonepublishers.com

FOR A COPY OF OUR CATALOG, CALL TOLL FREE: 877-900-BOOK, ext. 100